CHOOSING THERAPY

CHOOSING THERAPY

A Guide to Getting What You Need

Ilyana Romanovsky

ROWMAN & LITTLEFIELD
Lanham • Boulder • New York • Toronto • Plymouth, UK

Rowman & Littlefield
4501 Forbes Boulevard, Suite 200, Lanham, Maryland 20706
www.rowman.com

10 Thornbury Road, Plymouth PL6 7PP, United Kingdom

British Library Cataloguing in Publication Information Available

Library of Congress Cataloging-in-Publication Data
Romanovsky, Ilyana, 1982–
Choosing therapy : a guide to getting what you need / Ilyana Romanovsky.
pages cm
Includes bibliographical references and index.
ISBN 978-1-4422-2543-5 (cloth : alk. paper)—ISBN 978-1-4422-2544-2 (electronic)
1. Psychotherapy. 2. Psychotherapy—Evaluation. 3. Psychotherapist and patient. I. Title.
RC480.R66 2013
616.89'14—dc23
2013024915

♾™ The paper used in this publication meets the minimum requirements of American National Standard for Information Sciences Permanence of Paper for Printed Library Materials, ANSI/NISO Z39.48-1992.

Printed in the United States of America

CONTENTS

ACKNOWLEDGMENTS

I am grateful to my close friends who have supported me through this process and facilitated my writing. I also owe a great debt to my patients who have graced some of the pages of this book. Most of the cases I describe are true stories, although I have made significant modifications and changes to protect the identity of those who were so gracious to allow me to share snippets of their treatment. Also, the dialogue was my writing, not actual transcripts, and names and genders were changed to protect confidentiality of each patient's therapeutic experience.

In writing this book I also owe a great debt to my parents. Their enthusiasm, knowledge, wisdom, and most of all, emotional support helped me finish this project. They always know how to make me work while smiling.

INTRODUCTION

Try not. Do or do not. There is no try.

—Yoda

So you decided to give therapy a try. After many hours, weeks, or perhaps months of agonizing over whether therapy is the answer to your problem, you find yourself searching online for the best-rated shrink. "Is this guy experienced enough?" "Will my problems get resolved?" "How am I going to be able to pay for it?" "Can I even get through the hour with a perfect stranger?" This recognizable inner, scared voice in all of us assumes you are doing the right thing and simultaneously questions everything in the process.

Like any decision we make in life, beginning therapy involves mastering a large body of knowledge, navigating the thousands of therapists in the field and finding the right one, understanding different theoretical orientations, learning a variety of skills on how to be in therapy, and exploring one's innermost self with a complete stranger. The complexity of this journey is inadequately addressed in most books, if at all. Some folks are unfortunately stuck navigating this difficult process on their own, and leaving many decisions to chance. In this book, I address the experience of finding the right therapist and giving you the tools necessary to understand how aspects of different theoretical formulations affect the type of therapy that you receive. In the following chapters, I provide the knowledge to find the right therapist and introduce you to a new way of thinking through the process of therapy.

Over the years, many friends and family members, who wanted to begin therapy for various issues, asked the one question I heard most: "Who can I go and see for this issue?" For most people, the primary initial challenge of psychotherapy is understanding which type of therapy or therapist is better for a particular problem. Unlike any other field, psychology is something many people are interested in studying, and psychotherapy appeals to many, yet few divulge their personal experiences with therapy. Unfortunately, this defense handicaps people from hearing the necessary information on how to choose a good therapist and learning which particular therapeutic skills are best for intervening with specific problems. Regardless of therapeutic formulations and skill sets that therapists use in their practice, therapy itself is a very interpersonal experience between a therapist and a patient. There is no one-size-fits-all therapist and no average client. Learning how to give therapy is an art form, much like knowing how to receive it. The innermost, private world of a therapist is the most important guiding tool that therapists use when conducting sessions. Based on this aspect alone, it is possible to select a right therapist; however, like with anything else, it is also valuable to choose a therapist based on other professional skills, objectives, experience, and theoretical background. In this book I explore the experience of selecting the right therapist for you and if nothing else, make the entire journey of therapy understandable and easy— while keeping in mind the ultimate result of getting the most bang for your buck in personal psychotherapy.

Part I

Walking through the Door

I

PSYCHOTHERAPY EXPLAINED

He who has a why to live can bear almost any how.

—Friedrich Nietzsche

You decide to start therapy and you ask yourself, "How am I going to do this?" It is a common question to ask on the path of choosing the right therapist. But first thing first. To choose correctly, you have to know a little bit about the efficacy of psychotherapy, the importance of outcomes-informed care, and the different theoretical models therapists use when counseling patients. Let's start from the beginning.

Medicine and healing practices have existed since the origin of the human species and yet only recently did scientists question the efficacy of certain scientific disciplines. The one discipline that has received a great deal of scrutiny over the years is psychotherapy. Even as early as the 1950s, research claimed that certain therapeutic practices were not only unhelpful, but harmful to humans. About two decades later these original claims were disputed and showed that psychotherapy is effective as compared to the no-treatment control groups. Therefore, to address the first question of "Is psychotherapy effective?"—the answer is a resounding "yes." Now, what does this mean for you, a person thinking about beginning therapy? Well, for starters, giving yourself permission to trust in the process of therapy is a first step toward receiving positive benefits from therapy. After all, despite being willing to spend the money on therapy, questioning the efficacy of therapy could be a significant initial barrier toward progress.

When it comes to medicine, some treatments are clearly more effective than others. Looking through the latest research, you can quickly surmise that certain studies have better outcomes than others. It is easy to check the latest popular literature, scientific journals, or newspapers and discover which treatment is more effective for a specific ailment. What about psychotherapy? The next question many ask is: "Are some therapies more effective than others?" and if so, then "how do I find a therapist that will deliver a therapy that is most effective for my particular problem?"

Several years of research, including but not limited to many meta-analytical studies, concluded that generically, all treatments are about equally effective when delivered by therapists who believe in the treatment they are providing. There is, however, value in understanding the different types of treatment approaches. This reason has mainly to do with the type of therapy you would want to receive. This comes into play when considering long-term versus short-term psychotherapy, evidence-based versus nonevidence-based practices, and past versus present or future orientations. The therapist determines which key ingredients for successful treatment are delivered, as long as the therapy the therapist uses contains those specific ingredients.

The final and perhaps the most critical point to consider when choosing a therapist is expecting that psychotherapists be held accountable for the outcomes of their services. This accountability generally should not be delivered in the form of documentation stating that particular treatments were provided during the course of psychotherapy. Rather, this accountability has to come from the therapists themselves, knowing and having access to a data source containing information about the outcomes of the services they deliver. This component is crucial, as it allows therapists to have a self-correction mechanism throughout the course of the therapy. Therefore, when walking through the door initially, ask your therapist if he has a method for collecting outcomes data on his clients. Do not wait to ask this question, as it may be one of the most important questions to ask a psychotherapist. Ask about if you will be given forms or questionnaires to fill out at the end of each session, tracking and recording your individual progress in therapy. Take advantage of an opportunity to track your progress throughout the course of your therapy to benchmark your final outcomes versus your initial presenting data and concerns. Frankly, the odds of effective therapy delivery by any clinician without evidence of their outcomes are slim to none. Therefore, take advantage of outcomes-informed care, which is discussed further in later chapters.

Let us now embark on the journey of understanding what therapy is all about.

2

THEORIES OF PSYCHOTHERAPY

Show me a sane man and I will cure him for you.

—C. G. Jung

One of the most difficult things when becoming a therapist is choosing a particular theoretical orientation that helps guide work with clients. Beginning therapists often struggle with the decision as to which theory aligns most with their worldviews and how that theory will help them in their daily, therapeutic work. Once the process of choosing a particular framework is final, therapists devote a great deal of time learning how to orient sessions, adhering closely to the selected theory.

In the world of psychotherapy, therapists can consider several theories. For the purposes of this book, every theory in existence will not be discussed; however, it will be helpful to explain several major theories in the field and how these theories affect therapists' work. Because adherence to a particular framework guides the manner with which a therapist leads his or her sessions, this decision also affects the client, by way of learning how certain theoretical orientations resolve the nature of presenting problems. In light of all these factors, this book discusses the specifics of most major theories and gives relevant examples of how both a behaviorist and psychoanalyst would tackle mental health issues.

In the field of psychotherapy, therapists tend to choose from the popular, recognized frameworks. One of the most familiar is the psychoanalytic theory developed by its founding father, Sigmund Freud. Other approaches exist, such as: Adlerian, Jungian, existentialist, person-centered, Gestalt, cognitive-behavioral, reality based, transpersonal, and integrative. Again, the goal of this book is not to educate you about every major theoretical framework in existence, but to give you the necessary information of the more popular theoretical frameworks and how these frameworks guide the type of therapy you receive for your particular set of problems.

The history of psychoanalysis begins with Sigmund Freud. Psychoanalysis often involves techniques designed for uncovering hidden psychic processes over several years. Psychoanalytic work has evolved since then, now yielding variations of psychoanalysis. The classic techniques, however, are still employed by many therapists today. If you are considering sessions with a psychoanalyst, know that it is a long-term commitment. The aim of psychoanalysis is primarily to increase the clients' insights into themselves. A particular analyst may choose to work with a client on uncovering unconscious processes through the methods of interpretation, free association, and transference.[1] These fancy terms mean that your therapist will work with you on your roadblocks and resistances to uncover particular insights about yourself. This process is handled through continual analysis to achieve greater awareness into yourself and your problems.

When discussing specific intervention strategies as it touches on psychoanalysis, it is often a difficult topic to tackle, because psychoanalysis is largely based on free association. A client would take an hour to uncover deeply hidden thoughts or feelings toward the therapist, with the therapist often representing a close figure from a client's life such as a parent, sibling, or a child. This process involves the transfer of feelings—that is, "transference" from past relationships onto the psychoanalyst.

Consider this example. You seek out advice from a therapist concerning your anxiety issue. This anxiety is preventing you from completing tasks at home and around the office, and you finally decide to consult a professional. As it so happens, you land on the doorsteps of a psychoanalyst. In your initial session with Dr. X, you describe your present problem as well as the various avenues you have explored to wrestle with your problem. You tell Dr. X that you read several self-help books and had even taken yoga and tried meditation before, but your situation did not improve. You want Dr. X to spend a limited amount of time on this problem and explain that you are often out of town on business and would like this problem resolved quickly. This is a common scenario nowadays, as most people seek therapy in the hopes of getting rid of their problems immediately. The problem only arises, when Dr. X politely explains, after taking your history and $150 for the session, that his work requires more than just a few weeks. In return, you politely implore Dr. X to tell you what to do, maybe even complete a few homework assignments to expedite the process. You once again explain that you don't have years or months to peel away your defenses and your anxiety has to be dealt with now. After much back and forth, you and Dr. X agree that this type of therapy may not be a good fit, and once again, you feel defeated and lost in your search for the right therapist. In this scenario, the only winner is the present anxiety issue. One can argue brief forms of psychoanalysis exist; however, analysts, by definition, delve into the workings of the mind, beneath the surface of words, to reach the unconscious. This unfortunately takes years. If you are ready for long-term therapy, this is the perfect therapy for you. To avoid being discouraged from this type of therapy, Fisher and Greenberg[2] compiled close to two thousand individual research studies to highlight that Freudian theory has scientific merit and resiliency. Despite these affirmations, however, current critics of psychoanalysis argue that the length of treatment is a large limitation to this approach and briefer, more efficient models of treatment exist. When you decide to pursue psychoanalytic treatment, understand that the value of this path is not in its economics.

Let's take your anxiety problem to another therapist, an Adlerian. After the initial session with a psychoanalyst, you decide to try another therapist, Dr. Y. Your initial visit goes something like this:

Dr. Y: When you resolve your anxiety issue, what would you like to be able to do?

Patient: I haven't thought about it much, but I suppose I would like to be able to give more public presentations related to my research as well as be able to be more involved in my son's after school activities.

Dr. Y: Do you believe in yourself to resolve this issue of anxiety?

Patient: I don't know, Doc.

Dr. Y: When you were young, do you remember having big hopes for your life?

Patient: Certainly.

Dr. Y: It would appear to me that when you were younger, you had more courage and hope for yourself than now. If you know this, then you will leave this session remembering how important it is to be courageous, hopeful, and to a degree certain at being able to overcome life's problems, including this anxiety problem.

This brief exchange highlights a key point about Adlerian therapists. Adlerians use earlier recollections as an element of encouragement and motivation throughout the course of therapy.[3] The psychological process is tied to a client setting goals that are immediate as well as long term. Emotions are fueled during the therapeutic exchange, to help clients attain their goals. More specifically, change or in this case, resolution of anxiety happens due to a number of mechanisms at play. Insight is one of the key mechanisms of change, just as it is in psychoanalysis. Unlike psychoanalysis, however, insight is not the only ingredient present in the process of change. Adlerians help clients recognize their intentions in life and magnify those intentions by purposefully aggravating and challenging the person's internal dogma about what they are and are not capable of accomplishing. Encouragement is an essential element in therapy. Adlerians restore clients' faith in themselves by creating an awareness of their power to change when it comes to their problems.[4]

If you suddenly discover yourself taking a liking to this type of therapy, be prepared to take a long look at your lifestyle and analyze it with your Adlerian therapist. A classic example of Adlerian therapy is looking into your family, friends, or professional relationships, and analyzing yourself from the perspective of being an individual in the context of those relationships. This analysis happens by way of examining your upbringing and even birth order. The analysis can also take the form of looking into how you manage responsibility in your relationships and to whom you are normally accountable.

Adlerian theory has been validated as a therapeutic, rehabilitative model in the field of psychotherapy. The research to support the theory's applicability to individual, everyday problems has become internationally recognized and cross-culturally applicable. One of the issues, however, regarding Adlerian theory is its focus on examining individuals in terms of their relationships versus an emphasis on symptoms.[5] As it may be, Adlerians never look for symptoms and search for causes, but rather view problems as relational. Critics would argue still, that this lack of emphasis on symptoms demonstrates a lack in specific effectiveness of therapy as it touches on symptomatology that cannot be readily explained, such as schizophrenia or bipolar disorder. Therefore, in my opinion, if you are considering therapy with an Adlerian, the problems that are more effectively solved using the Adlerian framework are those that are in the context of general areas such as business or career, family, or friendships.

Is it possible to find a therapist who is more philosophical in her approach to therapy? Absolutely! I ask this question to introduce another psychological theory—the existential theory. Arising from the writings of Nietzsche, Kierkegaard, Camus, and Sartre, existentialism came into the forefront of psychology after World War II. Devastated by the brutalities of war, people turned to realism as an essential part of their existence. The process of change evolved from an implicit understanding that man had to face loneliness to transcend life. Only by being open about the raw, individual existence could men increase insight into their own being.[6]

Interestingly enough, although existentialism developed into a prominent theory, therapists have few techniques to use when working with clients. In fact, the therapist holds true to the notion that no two people are alike, no matter how similar the diagnoses. Every situation, person, encounter, and session are unique; therefore, no specific set of scientific procedures can be accurately applied to any single case. Listening to a client's story and finding meaning, awareness, and a larger perspective in the story becomes the sole focus of existential work. Clients would be encouraged to share their life journey, with the therapeutic lens set to uncover life's meaning and value. When in session, an existentialist would typically encourage clients to use the therapeutic relationship as a tool for learning, with the listener (i.e., the therapist) providing compassion and empathic, positive understanding. The therapist focuses on helping the client become more aware and stay aware in the moment.

Much like psychoanalysis, existential psychotherapy involves long-term commitment. Generally, the work focuses on realizing clients' full potential as it fits into their daily lives. This, however, is not the most practical form of therapy in existence today given the fast-paced development of insurance companies and limited resources. Existential counselors and therapists have dabbled in the pool of developing and providing brief therapy. However, this approach is often too intense for clients, as they are encouraged to deal with heavy issues such as death, isolation, anxiety, and meaning in a short time.

On a more positive note, existentialism is a relatable form of therapy today, given the advance of technology and the growing sense of isolation that more and more people experience. The electronic revolution makes it virtually impossible to go to work without carrying some sort of device such as a tablet, smartphone, or laptop, which by the way, have become so light and thin, you wonder if you grabbed it at all this morning in your rush to leave the house. In a culture that increasingly values detachment, many feel alienated and isolated. The full spectrum of disorders then is a direct result of this detachment and can be addressed through existential therapy. If you decide to undergo therapy with an existentialist after reading this brief overview, keep in mind that this type of approach involves long-term commitment and very little sound, scientific backup to its methods.[7]

In graduate school I was introduced to yet another theory of counseling psychology named person-centered theory (PCT). PCT is likely the most popular field of psychology and education. The theory was developed by Carl Rogers in the 1940s and has subsequently been known as "Rogerian theory." The key points to this type of therapy involve the patient relying fully on himself for autonomous development. A patient is encouraged to rely on his own experiences and the desire and ability to make positive changes. PCT therapists treat their clients with positive genuine regard, empathy, and trustworthiness. This type of therapy requires clients to complete the therapeutic work on their own, with minimal involvement from the therapist.[8] Consider an example below of a typical Rogerian approach to therapy.

A twenty-six-year-old female attends therapy for issues with substance abuse, three past arrests for shoplifting, and an eviction notice from her landlord for not paying rent. Many in our society would be quick to judge such a person and have little doubt in their mind that someone like that could not be trusted. The young female in our example would most likely recognize the lack of trust from others and have very little motivation to change her behaviors. A Rogerian therapist would begin by building the trustworthiness of the relationship between the two of them, and convey that trust to the client. A major part of the work in therapy will involve the therapist building that trust with the client through words and actions. Once this fundamental base is established, our client can begin to accept the ownership of her past mistakes and be motivated enough to grow into an honest and genuine person in her relationships with others.

From a Rogerian perspective, humans are always striving to be the best versions of themselves. This clearly becomes the biggest motivational force in therapy, based on conditions of autonomy and self-actualization. Our client would most likely be viewed as someone lacking self-control and desire to create and overcome her issues by many people's standards. If she had been led to therapy by a parent or a concerned friend, it is a safe bet to make that they would have tried to control her issues in the past and would have most likely had many conversations with her in regards to appropriate societal behaviors and norms. A Rogerian therapist, however, takes a different approach. Instead of focusing on our client's current "issues," the therapist emphasizes that the girl is actually working toward maximizing her potential and will continue regardless of others trying to interject and impose their own views on the situation. Our Rogerian therapist would send the girl home until next session, and talk to her loved ones about providing a safe place for her at home, without arguments or judgments. Ultimately, when the client begins to experience a safe, nonjudgmental environment at home, she will subsequently lower her defenses and work toward actualizing her true potential.

If you are entertaining the idea of starting therapy with a Rogerian, understand that this type of therapy is nondirective and is marked by minimal specific interventions from the therapist. Rogerians are required to be genuine and trustworthy of anyone who comes through their door seeking therapeutic services, rather than perform a rigid set of actions during sessions. If you require more guidance and homework during and after therapy, a Rogerian approach may not be for you. In many ways, PCT suffers most from its simplicity and lack of concrete interventions.[9] The supportive nature of PCT carries great concepts and ideals tied to human potential, however, these conditions alone are often not sufficient enough to guide clients toward meaningful change.

If you would be happy with a therapist who provides active listening, immediacy, and almost the exact reflection of content and feelings as you are sharing in therapy, then PCT may be right for you. Otherwise, keep reading through this chapter to find out if other therapies provide more activities and skills to give you the necessary boost you may benefit from.

If you are anything like me, you shop around and keep your options open for receiving services from medical or clinical specialists. With mental health services, I want to know that I am being understood. Throughout my training, I have been impressed by each mode of therapy, despite certain limitations. Every theoretical orientation has key aspects that allow its practitioners to understand their clients in their entirety. Given the complexity of our human behaviors, thoughts, emotions, and relationships, confusion and uncertainty are inevitable in therapy. That is why it is important to give a thoughtful commitment to a well-researched mode of therapy before making a snap judgment. Often our unfamiliarity with a particular profession or subject pushes us toward a premature conclusion, and it really does take courage to keep an open mind especially when allowing someone from the outside to help with your problems. This brings me to another mode of therapy, which may be easy to dismiss, but proven to be a well-researched aid in the therapeutic process.

Gestalt theory, originally developed with Fritz Perls, has influenced the course of therapeutic treatment all over the world. Gestalt counselors and therapists work with clients by looking at their "whole" being. The simple assumption behind Gestalt therapy is that people are capable of resolving their own problems, when they become fully aware of everything around them. Perhaps one of the more popular features of Gestalt psychotherapy is its holistic approach, versus an emphasis on pharmaceutical modes of treatment.

Research has demonstrated in the past the efficacy behind Gestalt psychotherapy. Studies have specifically examined the efficacy of this type of therapy as it touches on body issues related to body image and specific phobias. A meta-analysis study completed in 2004 by Strumpfel and Martin concluded that Gestalt therapy was effective when working with issues pertaining to substance abuse, chronic pain, and psychosomatic problems.[10] Interestingly, Gestalt therapy does not focus on client-related symptoms, but does address those symptoms through other means in the course of therapy.

How does Gestalt therapy work and what should you expect if you pursue therapy with a Gestalt practitioner? Well, unlike other modes of therapy discussed earlier in this chapter, Gestalt therapists have specific behavioral interventions that they encourage clients to use in sessions. These interventions are termed "experiments" and lead clients in their respective processes of self-awareness and self-discovery. These experiments involve dream work, where a client is asked to reenact a dream and play out parts of the dream. Other experiments include exaggeration of certain speech patterns or feelings in session to intensify the client's awareness of certain aspects of his posture, voice, or gestures. Perhaps the more popular Gestalt experiment involves asking the client to be his hand, fear, joy, or jealousy, and reenact that conversation. Another famous technique is an empty chair strategy designed to encourage clients to play a role in addition to himself. The client would speak for both parties, self, and the imagined party in the empty chair.[11] Gestalt clinicians are famous for their plethora of experiments intended to keep a client busy throughout the length of the session.

Research indicates that Gestalt therapy works best for those clients who are either overly expressive in their daily lives or overly intellectual and have difficulty with showing or identifying their feelings. Another piece to keep in mind about this type of therapy is that it will not provide you with a diagnosis at the end of the day.[12] If you like to know exactly where you fit in the *Diagnostic and Statistical Manual of Mental Disorders*, or DSM-5, you will not be categorized with a Gestalt therapist. Gestalt therapy is widely popular and well researched. It is generally applicable to a wide variety of disorders and can certainly be an unusual weekly fifty-minute discovery. This therapy generally focuses on the here and now versus examination of the past or future events and tends to deemphasize the cognitive components of therapy that are widely popularized in modern TV dramas and sitcoms. This type of therapy is yet another form of long-term therapy and can be incompatible with some clients wanting a more time-limited and brief psychotherapy.

What if you want a more time-limited therapy and are looking for someone in the area who might be insurance friendly and get you "patched-up" in a certain time? Keep reading through the end of this chapter, and I will introduce several short-term therapies that may be the right approach for you.

The first of the short-term therapies to discuss is named cognitive-behavioral therapy (CBT). The hyphen in the name reflects that this type of therapy involves both cognitive and behavioral approaches to helping clients resolve their issues. CBT considers the use of treatment interventions that encompass a range of methods, integrating cognitive as well as behavioral strategies. All cognitive interventions aim at influencing the thinking processes, which in turn influence behavioral and emotional processes. This alone is the major construct of cognitive-behavioral psychotherapy. Before delving into the treatment aspect, a cognitive-behavioral psychotherapist will conduct an assessment within two to three sessions. During these sessions, your therapist will focus on compiling a problem list of presenting issues, assigning a diagnosis, and establishing a treatment plan. Once this has been determined, the treatment phase will commence with a number of cognitive and behavioral interventions. Often, cognitive-behavioral therapists include the use of treatment manuals for the implementation of strategies that have been outlined and evaluated.

CBT is a brief approach to psychotherapy and most treatments of disorders such as anxiety or depression last between ten and twenty sessions. Sessions are held on the weekly basis keeping the psychotherapy process concrete and specific, and stressing homework assignments. Use of CBT is a collaborative venture between the therapist and the client, leaving little room for a passive passage of time. The therapist serves the role of providing the therapeutic structure and expertise at solving the client's problems. The process itself requires teamwork, with the client playing an active role in and outside sessions. Common intervention strategies might include Socratic questioning to dispute faulty or unhelpful beliefs about self or others, or certain behavioral strategies such as reinforcement of helpful behaviors, extinction of certain problematic behaviors, or even the use of environment to cue behaviors. The following exchange highlights the cognitive restructuring that often plays a role in CBT:

Therapist: You told me that you believe that you are worthless and will not amount to anything.

Patient: I do. I always mess up and make mistakes in my work.

Therapist: Can you think of anyone that you know that doesn't make mistakes?

Patient: I guess not. I guess everyone makes mistakes.

Therapist: Does that mean that everyone is worthless?

Patient: I see your point. I guess I can be less critical of myself.

This particular exchange between the therapist and the client shows examples and questions used to guide the client to the conclusion that her initial statement may be faulty and inaccurate. The inductive method is essential to CBT, simply because it forces clients to think critically and scientifically through their beliefs and problems. Clients are taught to think about their thoughts as statements that can be questioned, as opposed to facts that do not require any verification. Cognitive-behavioral therapists guide their clients to confront the evidence for their maladaptive beliefs and test their assumptions about themselves and others.[13] A case from my own clinical practice illustrates how CBT can be used in treatment with severe mental illness:

CASE STUDY I

One of my patients with psychosis met the criteria for schizophrenia and had a five-year history of mental health problems. Patient was prescribed antipsychotic medications in combination with other drugs, all of which he took with no exception. Embracing the cognitive behavioral module of treatment, I was able to identify that my patient's concerns were around hearing voices and believing that there was an active conspiracy against him. Working together for months, my patient and I initially prioritized specific and measurable goals. In regard to voices, my patient and I set an initial goal to use a percentage rating to track changes in control over voices, as well as distress caused by the voices. Even if frequency was left unaffected, my patient could still feel like he was making meaningful progress if the amount of control over voices increased. My patient was convinced that his voices came from a higher power, which were accompanied by a string of physical sensations in which he felt that the voices were compelling him to say and do things. The possibility that his voices were a symptom of mental illness is something that had to be brought up slowly. The work included working out metacognitive beliefs that thoughts and voices can be just that, thoughts and voices. Choosing to ignore the voices did not mean that one is responsible for whatever the voices were saying, and certainly did not imply that my patient had to act on the voices. The idea that my patient had a disorder became more apparent to him when he had ignored the voices several times during the course of behavioral experiments and still found himself unpunished and alive. All interpretations were considered in great detail, and additional evidence for and against each interpretation had been specifically written out. During one of our sessions, my patient was highly animated, snapping his words off and pointing, while discussing his fears about the conspiracy. "By sneezing, my coworker let me know that I was lazy and deliberately sneezed to tell me how he felt about my work." This statement fit with my patient's presentation that those around him are deliberately trying to send him a message or hurt him in some way.

"So it sounds like your colleague at work is involved in a conspiracy against you and by sneezing, he is indirectly accusing you of being lazy, which makes you upset."

"Yeah, that's pretty much the situation."

"If you wanted to change the way you felt about this situation, what would you need to do?"

"I could go on about my day and learn to ignore the sneezing."

"Are there other possible explanations for why your colleague may be sneezing?"

"Well, he could be getting over a cold, or there is the chance that he could be allergic to something in the office. Sometimes I sneeze when I am allergic to something."

"What is the possibility that any of these reasons could apply in this case? Does it seem likely that one of the reasons could be true and your colleague is not criticizing your work, but is simply allergic or getting over a cold?"

"There is a slight possibility that he is sick or allergic, and his sneezing has nothing to do with me."

My patient and I examined specific evidence around the conspiracy theory over the next few months. Our sessions focused on breaking down the facts and considering possibilities for certain events occurring. The distress associated with persecutory beliefs decreased for my patient over the course of four sessions and it was done partly because he was willing to consider the evidence and believe other interpretations of the events. This resulted in a reduction of his convictions from 85 percent to 10 percent and a dramatic decrease in distress ratings.

CBT has been developed and used with clients who have a wide variety of issues and clinical problems. There is also a great deal of research to support the efficacy of CBT, which is currently used to treat schizophrenia, bipolar disorder, anxiety, depression, panic disorder, attention-deficit hyperactivity disorder (ADHD), behavioral issues, and many other disorders. CBT is a therapeutic approach that is diverse enough that it can be applied to a multitude of diagnoses and clinical issues. The following case study illustrates treatment of depression using CBT:

CASE STUDY 2

My patient was suffering from depression and had a long history of therapeutic treatment prior to beginning CBT. As my patient and I commenced our work together, I asked her to make a list of concerns that she wanted to work through in treatment. I also asked for the list of concerns to be in order of severity. It was important to focus on how my patient was feeling during the times when stressors and concerns were particularly heightened. My patient took the time to name instances in which her feelings were most severe and the thoughts that accompanied those feelings. A rather important piece of therapy was to understand how the patient had coped with her difficulties in the past, and what had helped her mood to be more positive in those situations. As we continued to develop the list of concerns, I also wanted to be able to understand my patient's understanding of her own difficulties. Did she attribute her difficulties to her own internal will power or were those difficulties outside of her realm of control? For example, when I asked my patient about the origin of her depressed feelings, she attributed them to her traumatic childhood. In this particular case, it became important to delve deeper into the meaning that my patient had attached to those early experiences. Had my patient not learned the necessary skills to deal with life's challenges or had she been defeated and scarred by certain early traumas, that it would be difficult for her to conceptualize she was capable of change.

The next phase of treatment involved a formulation of an accurate case conceptualization for treatment. My patient reported an array of cognitive distortions that fueled her depression. Some of these distortions involved hopelessness and not seeing the light at the end of the tunnel. Other distortions involved magnification, continually berating herself for the inability to make any type of decision, as well as personalization of negative events (i.e., thinking that she was responsible for her own misfortunes, and identifying her past as the origin for her inaction). I asked my patient to think about how often she exhibited her unhelpful thinking, and the situations that occurred in which that type of thinking was triggered. My patient's early childhood experiences had taught her to think of herself as incapable, flawed, and defective. Sessions were centered on those core beliefs, asking her to describe those beliefs in detail to understand the meanings and associations that they had for my patient. Once those details were gathered, only then could I work with my patient to refute those maladaptive beliefs and teach her to look at them as behavioral traits, as opposed to ingrained aspects of her personality. In the months that followed, my patient was asked to identify and evaluate her maladaptive thoughts. She was encouraged to reflect on her thinking, her emotions, and also to look at situations that triggered her depression. She dutifully kept a diary of her thoughts, and practiced identifying automatic thoughts that perpetuated her depressogenic schemas. As triggers were more evident, we began using rational responding in sessions to evaluate the validity of her thoughts. I asked my patient a number of simple questions to challenge her underlying beliefs. These questions ranged from: "What is the evidence for and against your belief?" "Is there an alternative explanation or a more helpful way of looking at things?" Was it true for example that the patient's daughter did not care about her feelings and was only preoccupied with making her life miserable?

A cognitive-behavioral therapist establishes a plan to work with patients in such a way as to focus on developing an understanding of the role thinking has on a particular situation. Patients learn to challenge and identify thoughts that trigger depression, as well as patterns of thoughts categorized as unhelpful, that bring about feelings of angst, anxiety, or frustration related to depression. Then the primary task of a cognitive-behavioral therapist is to demonstrate that thoughts, feelings, and behaviors are interrelated, and that psychotherapy will work through changing maladaptive thoughts for maximization of positive, therapeutic outcomes.

The union of cognitive-behavioral therapists is a strong force in modifying and implementing the theory to make it applicable and effective when treating a number of diagnoses. However, psychotherapists who are big proponents of psychoanalysis continue to object and state that CBT lacks in its emphasis on the unconscious processes when it comes to treatment of clinical disorders.[14] Additionally, CBT does not stress exploring the client's past issues and concerns, but focuses on the "here and now" to determine specific unhelpful thoughts, beliefs, and behaviors that can be modified to ameliorate symptoms. Being a cognitive-behavioral therapist, I have little criticism when it comes to this particular theoretical approach. With that out in the open, I suggest exploring this type of therapy as it is efficient and successful in treating most disorders. The numerous interventions used require a specific and concrete approach to treatment that is limited in time and efficient. Depending on the case and the individual, this type of treatment allows many to lead functioning, balanced lives without having to spend a fortune in therapy or commit to a decade of resolving one's issues.

Another short-term therapy available is called reality therapy. This type of therapy originated with William Glasser and developed mainly in settings such as psychiatric hospitals and correctional institutions. Glasser developed this theory after finding that psychoanalysis did not necessarily achieve the goal of making people change their behaviors.

In fact, reality therapy stresses that humans are responsible for their own behaviors and cannot blame the environment, upbringing, or the past on their current set of issues. Glasser emphasized that everyone always has choices and that people have an option to choose how they will behave. Therefore, the goals of reality psychotherapy are measured through behavioral changes and not merely through gaining insight into one's problems.[15]

The main theory that underlies reality therapy is called choice theory. Choice theory presupposes that human beings are born with needs and the difference between what humans want and need is the source of human behaviors. The goals of this therapy are to help people satisfy their needs.[16] These goals are written down and generally follow the criteria of being measurable, simple, immediate, controlled by the client, and attainable. In the past, this type of therapy received a great deal of criticism for being so pointed and problem oriented, that it took away from the gradual process of change that is found in traditional long-term psychotherapy. Proponents of this type of therapy, however, do not apologize for its efficient and organized approach to counseling and put a great deal of value on its reliability and effectiveness.

A typical reality therapy session involves your therapist allowing time for silence, encouraging clients to self-evaluate. Other tools used include repetitive questions such as "How did it work out for you?" or "What impact did your behaviors have at the time?" or "Did making these choices help you accomplish your goals in the past?" Such questions reinforce to clients the assumption that responsibility is on their shoulders for the choices they make in life. Among other interventions is the use of optimism to convey to clients their future success and even implementation of consequences that often occurs in correctional settings.[17] Specific interventions are the essence of reality therapy and are based on discussions of client wants, needs, and perceptions, as well as a discussion of behavioral direction, evaluations, and future planning.

Like any theory, reality therapy is not without its critics. Many believe that for clients to achieve any lasting, meaningful change, they have to acquire insight into their lives, including all past events. This insight is gained through weekly discussions of past conflicts and traumas. Yet another drawback is the concrete, simple language of reality therapy, leaving some critics arguing that it may be too simplistic for practice.[18] With all these limitations however, proponents of this therapy rely on the research to back up the measured effectiveness of this type of counseling. Lawrence, for example, used reality therapy to test its effectiveness in a group modality with clients struggling with developmental disorders.[19] After only six sessions, group members showed marked increase in self-determination, empowerment, and autonomy as compared to the control group who did not receive reality therapy. Even though more research can be conducted to validate reality therapy, its widespread interest and use is undeniable. Reality therapy is a cross-cultural method to treatment and has been widely accepted with diverse populations in Asian, South African, Middle-Eastern, and European countries. Evidence also points to its effectiveness with a variety of issues such as eating disorders, marriage counseling, career satisfaction, self-esteem, and aging related difficulties.[20] If you find this therapy appealing, research more about the therapy's effectiveness as it relates to your particular set of issues. Overall, this type of therapy is brief and solution focused, and if time spent in therapy is a concern, reality therapy can definitely help you acquire necessary skills to manage your problems.

The last theory that I will mention in this chapter is called rational emotive behavior therapy (REBT). This is yet another form of brief, short-term psychotherapy, with Albert Ellis as the founding father of the theory. As a young man and an innovator in the field of psychotherapy, Ellis experimented with different types of therapies, including psychoanalysis. By the early 1950s, REBT was born. The basic tenets of this theory are deeply rooted in philosophy, as Ellis was well versed in both psychology and philosophy. In fact, REBT grew from writings and teachings of Epictetus, who held the belief that people disturb themselves not by interacting and stumbling against events or situations in life, but by the type of meanings they make of the obstacles they stumble against. Ellis formed this new theory on the assumption that human beings have an innate ability to irrationality, regardless of upbringing, education, or life experiences. Ellis argued that at some point every human has the capacity to think illogically and irrationally, and REBT is designed to increase people's happiness by building on more rational thinking and cutting down on the emotional distress.[21]

The basic premise of REBT is that this type of psychotherapy is psychoeducational and puts the responsibility of thinking rationally, flexibly, and logically on the client. The focus of therapy is on the disturbed emotions and behaviors leading to unhappiness. As a result of this type of thinking and psychotherapeutic approach, REBT therapists and counselors are very involved and active in therapy. The therapeutic relationship begins to thrive from the minute clients choose to walk through the door and establish goals for change. Moreover, clients actually leave the first session with some insight and hope for enhancing their ability to handle everyday issues.

Ellis developed a conceptual model of REBT that guides the process of change. This model is known as the ABC Model and stands for activating event, beliefs, and emotional or behavioral consequences. The ABC model posits that problems are encountered because there is a block or trigger that prevents people from accomplishing their goals. This activating event or trigger is then misinterpreted or attributed negative meaning by the individuals experiencing the trigger. The misinterpretations develop into negative core beliefs that result in negative emotional or behavioral consequences. For example, a client seeks therapy for his fear around germs and thoughts of getting AIDS. The patient reasons that if he comes into contact with anything "public" such as public restrooms, door handles, or even shaking hands, he translates this into him acquiring AIDS. The attributed interpretation of the event/trigger (A) "touching a public phone" elicits the mistaken belief (B) that our patient will acquire AIDS. As a consequence (C), the patient feels anxious, worried, and paranoid every time he comes into contact with a public item. This basic model serves as a basis for REBT, which then guides its treatment.

REBT is replete with its set of interventions for many types of mental health issues. Some of these exercises involve behavioral interventions, which play an important role in helping clients reach their therapeutic goals. Other interventions involve shame-attacking exercises to help clients stop degrading themselves, along with role-playing, didactic disputes, and emotive interventions. Overall, REBT is applied widely to a variety of mental disorders including anxiety, depression, obsessive-compulsive disorder, panic disorder, agoraphobia, borderline personality disorder, and others.[22] The experiential exercises used in REBT can be applied in an individual one-on-one session as well as group and classroom settings. REBT targets teaching clients new skills that they can use in the future to explore problematic areas in their behaviors or emotions.

Having stated before that I am a cognitive behavioral therapist and enjoy practicing this type of therapy, I believe REBT and CBT help people address their issues in a time efficient manner as opposed to other therapies. I also find the importance in recognizing that even the most effective therapies alone are sometimes ineffective, because not everyone wants to let go of their irrational beliefs and self-defeatist ways. Research has shown in the past that many disorders are best targeted through brief, short-term therapies in addition to pharmacotherapy. Therefore, it is difficult to address the question of how effective a particular type of therapy will be for a specific set of issues. Rather, it is more time worthy to consider how ready you are for the process of change and how hard you are willing to work at resolving your issues outside of the regularly scheduled therapy sessions.

Initially, everyone who has considered therapy at one time or another has struggled with the "how to find the right therapist." Generally consumers struggle to link theory to the type of issues they have or even the type of therapy they would consider. When you start out seeing a psychotherapist, the theoretical and practical aspects of your issues most likely reside in two separate areas of your brain. If you do not have a graduate degree in the field, it is difficult to know which type of therapy to consider when beginning the search for a therapist. After many hours, months, and even years in therapy, some clients might feel that there is something wrong with them, in that they still haven't figured out how to resolve their issues. One way to avoid this trap is by researching the available types of therapies out there and thinking through what you may want out of your therapist. Asking the right questions such as "Do I want an active therapist or a passive one?" "Do I want to be doing extra work outside the sessions?" or "What is the amount of sessions I would be comfortable with to target a specific problem?" are all good questions to ask when considering the ins and outs of therapy. This chapter gave a brief overview of the types of therapies available. Remember, not all psychotherapy theories and theorists have been included here, just those that are the most available counseling approaches. With more research, or even reading this chapter, you'll easily become a competent and successful consumer. Make a point of familiarizing yourself with the different theories of practice, and you will be pleased with the result of your time spent in therapy.

3

INTERVENTIONS IN PSYCHOTHERAPY

If you want to conquer the anxiety of life, live in the moment, live in the breath.

—Amit Ray

Recently, patients come into my office and ask about mindfulness-based approaches to psychotherapy. It is interesting that patients are asking about mindfulness, not me introducing the subject. Living and practicing in the state of California, mindfulness has a big following, with centers set up with the commitment to develop trainings, resources, and mindfulness awareness in the communities. Mindfulness also has a place in psychotherapy, and two approaches specifically have been recognized and validated with empirical research to substantiate treatment.

Mindfulness refers to a state of being fully present, in the present moment and comes to us from ancient spiritual traditions. Within Buddhism, mindfulness is an integral practice into awareness and movement away from suffering. It is also integral to being human. Mindfulness is neither religious in its elements and practice, nor is it esoteric. Mindfulness is rather a practice and a way of approaching life that encompasses certain attitudes such as acceptance, patience, nonjudgment, and compassion for self and others. Mindfulness is an awareness that emerges when we pay attention to experiences with a spirit of acceptance. This practice incorporates three broad components: awareness, attitude, and understanding of human vulnerability. How does this tie into psychotherapy, you may ask? Well, in the previous chapter, I introduced a theoretical approach to psychotherapy, CBT. The other subcategory of CBT is mindfulness-based cognitive behavioral therapy (MBCT). Mindfulness meditation is the basis for MBCT that also has roots in CBT.

Prior to the development of MBCT, evidence-based psychotherapy treatment included CBT combined with pharmacotherapy. MBCT was first developed as a cost-effective relapse prevention approach for treatment of unipolar depression.[1] The approach asks what makes people prone to depressive relapse and which skills from the cognitive-behavioral model can be transferred and applied using MBCT. As a particular patient continues to experience depressive relapse episodes, less and less stress is required to provoke another episode. This is mainly due to the internal thinking structure of the person experiencing depression. The internal belief system fuels the negative thinking pattern and the patient is once again vulnerable to future depression. Most importantly, everyone is prone to lows in mood; however, if a person has a history of depression, the low periods become moments of heightened vulnerability to relapse.

In particular, two specific thinking patterns are unhelpful in perpetuating the cycle of depression. One such pattern is called rumination, which is a repetitive, brooding, self-judgmental, and critical way of thinking. A person spends hours preoccupied with the desire to fix whatever emotional or situational challenges are in the way to happier mood states. A second unhelpful thinking pattern is avoidance—an attempt to not think about an upsetting situation or deal with challenging emotions. During depressive episodes in particular, this pattern is repeated and the connection to utilize these thinking styles is strengthened as the person continues back to what is "known" versus attempting to change these patterns.

In regards to how CBT plays a role in MBCT, readers should understand specific key points that people who have engaged in CBT treatment learn to prevent future depressive episodes. CBT teaches patients to work with the content of their thoughts, bringing awareness to their thinking patterns as well as gradually exposing patients to change the relationship they have with their thoughts and feelings. Through the process of engagement in CBT, patients begin to view their difficult thoughts and feelings as passing events that may not reflect the factual realities of the moment. In essence, CBT teaches patients to take a decentered approach to their thinking, and then disengage from the emotionally intense entanglements of their inner world. The ability to remove oneself from one's thoughts and examine the rationality of those thoughts is precisely the intent of MBCT. Consequently, the practice of MBCT focuses on the awareness of the moment and all of the thoughts and feelings that come up in that moment.[2] MBCT then guides patients to relate to their thoughts as passing aspects of awareness as opposed to reality itself. Once that process is strengthened through experience and practice, patients can learn to recognize their thoughts as thoughts alone and not as facts.

How does MBCT work? The therapist's goal is to facilitate patients' ability to step out of their ruminative and brooding thinking processes, recognize and catch body-related sensations associated with depressive thinking styles, access new ways of thinking and engage in the experience, and avoid negative emotions. In this way, an MBCT therapist leads a patient toward symptom management. Now, how do these steps really work?

Any human is only able to sustain attention for a certain time period and process a limited amount of information coming in. Therefore, when patients attempt to focus on particular aspects of their experience, such as rumination on negative thoughts, they are also blocking out other information processing that could take place in their stead. Rather than pursuing the issue, and attempting to solve whatever challenge a patient perceives in his life, an MBCT therapist would encourage the patient to learn ways to direct his attention elsewhere, on a different type of experience. Thoughts are simply acknowledged as a series of processes that occur simultaneously with all the other processes, such as external events or body sensations.[3] Patients are then taught to attend to those thoughts that they want more of in their field of awareness. Through repeated practice and skill building, patients learn to recognize negative thinking patterns, and rather than being driven by those automatic thoughts, they instead learn how to respond differently to their thoughts.

MBCT focuses on revealing to patients, through the process of therapy, how a mind can be a creature of habit. Over years of certain experiences, we learn to react and think in certain ways. Patients begin to recognize that minds are not always our best friend and at times run on autopilot, caught up in ruminative and to an extent, destructive cycles. Patients learn to identify these cycles, tune into their triggers, and maintain a general awareness of their cognitive and behavioral patterns that lead to depression. The shift toward a more mindful mode of thinking involves paying attention to the present moment and relating to depression differently from what experience and habit have dictated. The new shift in thinking can involve recognizing that a particular moment or experience is not defining and can be seen as an aspect of an experience that occurs in the moment. This can create a subtle shift in perception, from viewing an experience as an all-encompassing, never-ending pattern of defeat to identifying an experience as just that, one experience. In this manner, patients learn to not acknowledge things as heavily and look at the moment through a more or less decentered lens. Rather than being caught up in the thinking, it becomes possible to gain a much broader perspective, keeping in mind that there are other experiences that will ultimately define another moment.

The last and final area taught through MBCT is the experience of turning toward emotions as opposed to away from them. Emotions can be pleasant, unpleasant, or not evoke any feelings at all, but the patient learns how to tolerate all emotions, regardless of origin or color. Patients learn to accept their experiences through compassion and a nonjudgmental attitude. This again is another shift that teaches patients to process experiences by deliberately facing difficult emotions and circumstances. Most people spontaneously experience moments in the present without being caught up in the firestorm that can be the mind. For many, however, a fog or preoccupation with the negative surrounds the everyday moment. The rationale for mindfulness is the foundation of MBCT, which rests on the practice of enabling patients to intentionally disengage from the autopilot, bring back attention to the present, and open up a solution pool of options. Unfortunately, rumination happens outside human awareness and the effects on emotional experiences can be catastrophic. One clinician described the experience of the autopilot as getting on a bus and missing all the stops along the way without realizing what is happening. The style of processing experiences in such a way becomes so habitual that patients can spiral downward quickly into depressed mood states, without actually knowing exactly what brought them into those states. Thus, MBCT provides the skills necessary for patients to "catch" their minds before they miss all the bus stops, directing their thoughts and attention to those aspects they want more of (i.e., positive, balanced thoughts). The diversion of attention is frequently done by asking patients to focus on any sensory experiences that they may be aware of in the moment, and rather than analyzing or making judgments about their thoughts, patients learn to take on the attitude of acceptance and compassion (i.e., "There goes my mind jumping to the worst possible case scenario again"). Thus, MBCT offers a way to relate to the present moment in a friendly and noncritical manner.

To give readers a more practical understanding of MBCT if considering this therapy, the general shape of the program is anywhere between eight to ten weeks. The length of sessions will vary depending on the practicing clinician, but can go up to two-and-half-hours long per session.[4] Much like CBT, patients have structured homework assignments requiring them to practice skills learned in sessions. The homework can be a daily forty-five-minute meditation and possibly some monitoring of body sensations during the meditation practice. Generally, therapy begins by teaching patients meditation with an emphasis on internal experiences, gradually bringing focus to processes happening within. As therapy progresses, patients learn to focus meditations with an application to life's challenges, incorporating more external shifts in awareness.

From week one in MBCT, patients learn to conduct a body scan, which is a mindful movement of awareness to each part of the body. Following this introduction, patients learn a mindfulness scan at home, subsequently recording and discussing their experiences in the following session. Throughout the teaching process, an MBCT clinician will additionally introduce didactic components, linking experiential learning to whichever challenges patients bring into the weekly sessions. Patients also learn a breathing exercise that can last anywhere from three to five minutes that supports the connection between mindfulness and didactic processing.[5] Within all of this, the interaction between a clinician and a patient becomes important, built on safety and trust. Patients learn to process events through a cognitive-behavioral perspective, while simultaneously incorporating the "awareness of the moment" into every session.

The intention of MBCT is to teach patients to incorporate mindfulness techniques in everyday life. Formal mindfulness practice in therapy becomes vital in giving patients a taste for what they are cultivating within themselves to address everyday worries and concerns. Detailed exploration of the effects of intentionally bringing in mindfulness practice can facilitate patients using these techniques to deliberately manage symptoms of anxiety and depression. As with any new skill, the integration of mindfulness practice into daily life does not happen spontaneously, and must be a conscious effort made on the part of the patient.

Also, other therapies are modeled after MBCT. These therapies are somewhat modified to fit the needs of the specific clinical groups in treatment. The new therapies have emerged only recently; therefore more evidence is necessary to conclude on the efficacy of their practices.

One of the emerging therapies is mindfulness-based eating awareness training and was developed in the effort to treat individuals with binge eating disorder and obesity. The therapy includes guided eating meditations to target issues of body image, weight, shape, and appetite. The framework of the therapy conceptualizes overeating as a direct result of a deregulation of mood, cognitions, and behaviors. Mindfulness training teaches patients to pay attention to their automatic thoughts and examine their belief systems, and thus change some of the patterns associated with reactivity. Many guided meditations incorporate food in sessions to teach participants techniques for mindful eating practices. A simple exercise of eating a slice of apple, while paying attention to thoughts and feelings facilitates the process of awareness to target emotional or reactive eating patterns. The therapy then progresses to challenging foods such as cakes and cookies, and finally a full buffet with the practice of making mindful food choices. This type of therapy additionally has components rooted in body work; however, they are minimal compared with traditional MBCT.[6]

Another emerging mindfulness-based therapy is named mindfulness-based relationship enhancement. This type of therapy attempts to develop relationships of couples who are happy, but are willing to look at areas that can be improved. The practical aspects of the therapy involve exercises in dyads, guiding partners to focus on channeling feelings of kindness toward one another. Kindness work is a big piece of this therapy in general and is often combined with other exercises to strengthen the nature of interventions used. Mindfulness-based relationship enhancement additionally places emphasis on listening skills, as well as communicational patterns to transfer healthy interactions into couples' daily lives. The therapy additionally involves some yoga exercises, mindful touch, and intimacy building. Overall, the therapy focuses on building healthy and strong relationships.[7]

Other mindfulness-based therapies are targeting relapse prevention around addiction treatment. Mindfulness-based relapse prevention integrates mindfulness along with the principles of CBT for substance abuse. The architects of the theory hypothesized that mindfulness could be integrated into relapse prevention to help participants feel and observe the moment, as opposed to a lifetime commitment to sobriety. Mindfulness-based relapse prevention therapy teaches specific skills to cope with urges and cravings. In recently published research, this therapy has been successfully implemented with patients struggling with alcohol and drug use issues, as well as with patients receiving treatment for smoking cessation.[8] Because the therapy is relatively new, more research is required to investigate the efficacy of the therapy.

Turning to other therapies that incorporate mindfulness, but stem from different theoretical roots, is dialectical behavioral therapy (DBT). Dialectical behavioral therapy was developed by Marsha Linehan, specifically as a therapy for treatment for borderline personality disorder. This therapy was later broadened and adapted for treatment of various other disorders. The central tenet of the therapy is acceptance as well as change. As part of the therapy techniques, DBT teaches formal mindfulness practices, although mindfulness exercises are typically much shorter than the formal mindfulness awareness training. Participants learn practical skills to target one's goals using mindfulness strategies to achieve them. The modules focus on the breath, body, emotional regulation, and distress tolerance. Patients are encouraged to attend completely to the present moment, as well as to act with spontaneity and without self-judgment. A large body of research supports the effectiveness of mindfulness training using the DBT approach, along with a robust clinical effectiveness for treatment of borderline personality disorder.[9]

Mindfulness-based interventions are an emerging new field that was developed for and is applied to a broad range of disorders and populations. The development of these interventions is quite exciting, potentially opening up unlimited possibilities for its application. The danger, however, is that mindfulness-based practices have a possibility of being changed, given the great variety of clinicians and trainings that are available. By far the biggest concern is that mindfulness will soon be far removed from its original Buddhist roots given the watered down approaches of all available therapies which use mindfulness-based practices. Readers should be aware of the plethora of therapies and modalities available in the field for intervention with each specific diagnosis or issue. We can only do so from a deeply informed position, drawing from both experience and evidence-based research.

Acceptance and commitment therapy (ACT) was first developed as an alternative to CBT that is based on the idea of learning how to decrease unhelpful, negative cognitions and emotions. ACT is rooted in the practice of behaviors despite negative or aversive thoughts and emotions. Therefore, a clinician who practices ACT will not teach a patient to change her unhelpful thoughts through cognitive restructuring methods, but rather accept those thoughts. ACT suggests the possibility of different approaches to addressing symptoms and distress. This is based on knowing that human distress is unavoidable given certain life's circumstances. Thus, instead of finding ways to decrease the frequency of certain thoughts and feelings, another approach is to accept the distress. The roots of this practice do not deviate much from advice a parent or a grandparent might give growing up: "Bear the burden and move forward." ACT teaches patients to accept their experience as it is, as opposed to what their minds might say their experience should be. [10]

The premise of ACT is rather simple. What we tell ourselves at times, if not frequently, translates into a certain type of behavior. For example, if Mitch lost his job, he may frame his experience in the following manner: "Men who have jobs are providers for their families. Men who do not have jobs cannot provide for their families, and are therefore inadequate. If I no longer have a job I am inadequate." If a patient is depressed, the cognition goes a step further to: "If I feel inadequate all the time, then I am nothing." As a result, Mitch may fall into a depressed state and lack the motivation necessary to look for jobs. The process described here highlights the common occurrence of the human brain jumping to tenuous conclusions based on the exaggerated idea or perceptions of what "should" be. Over time, people learn arbitrary ways of evaluating themselves based on those perceptions or beliefs—and they then hold them as absolute facts. For example, Julie might consider herself "unlovable" because she does not have a partner. "Not having a partner means that you are undesirable and unlovable" according to one of Julie's beliefs. Much in the same way, Peter may evaluate himself as weak for needing therapy, because "depressed people are weak" and Peter is depressed. Because our human experience is framed in words and language, people learn to bring significance to every thought based on nothing more than a feeling or a perceived idea.

Because these perceived ideas are not disputed in our daily living practice, we accept them as how the world truly is. Thoughts and beliefs begin to override direct experience, even when direct experience is in opposition to those thoughts and beliefs. Soon enough beliefs turn into rules and humans learn to live by the rules they set up. If you ask a patient at that moment how helpful his rules are, the answer is almost always invariably the same: "Not very helpful at all." What does ACT do then in terms of treatment? A clinician practicing this therapeutic approach will disrupt the maladaptive thinking processes by teaching a patient acceptance techniques, followed by what is known as cognitive diffusion, values work, and commitment strategies.[11]

Let's start with acceptance. The word acceptance can mean many things. In the words of our elders, it could mean to grind your teeth and move forward no matter how badly you may feel in the process. The running theme of ACT, however, is not to accept the process and soldier on. Rather, ACT involves a willingness to experience the distressing thoughts and emotions that drive the behaviors associated with certain values and beliefs. Therefore, instead of running away from negative emotions, acceptance is the experiential process of moving toward the negative. To describe ACT, take, for example, an emotional regulation technique that involves holding ice chips in both hands. As patients curl their fingers over the ice, the sensations that they generally report are the coldness and stiffness in their muscles as they keep clutching the ice. Additionally, other sensations may involve the mild burning associated with holding the ice until it melts. Patients learn, rather unexpectedly, that their one constant thought will not be that they will lose their hands to frostbite, but that sensations and thoughts will change and worries will come and go.[12] The experience teaches that noting the thoughts as the sensations persist as mere thoughts can be helpful. Holding the ice conveys the understanding that sometimes as we move in a certain direction and encounter setbacks, we might experience pain and distress. ACT then imparts psychological acceptance of the understanding that distress is a normal part of progress and, at times, humans cannot move closer to what they value, unless they experience the distress.

From an ACT perspective, introducing cognitive work into the treatment process is the next step since humans have a tendency to use language and to either magnify or minimize events that are especially emotionally charged. ACT uses a technique called diffusion to undercut the processes responsible for any cognitive distortions. As described with an earlier example, distress and discomfort remain; however, a patient puts things in perspective and accepts the distress while continuing to move toward realistic and measurable goals in life. Diffusion strategies cannot be expected to fully and permanently rationalize emotionally laden events, but the evaluation of those experiences can be expected to improve with acceptance and diffusion strategies.

All learning happens in the present moment. Using ACT, patients learn to track their behaviors in the moment and tune into their reactions. At times, patients are easily carried away from the moment by getting lost in thought. For example, you may be walking down the street and notice a beautiful necklace in the window of one of the stores. Your thoughts jump to evaluations of the necklace: "necklace," "expensive," "gorgeous." Soon enough your thoughts are taking you along for a trip: "I wonder what it would be like to own such a beautiful necklace"; "I could show up at my reunion wearing that necklace"; "My classmates would think that I made it in life if I wore something like that." As you are taking this cognitive trip, you notice a boy on a bike directly behind you, who has been trying to pass you for the last few minutes, and is vigorously ringing his bell. In the few minutes that he was waiting, the boy grew impatient and started to yell. Unfortunately, getting lost in thought does not always have pleasant consequences, and it does benefit to stay in the present moment. This is not to say that we should never fantasize or take cognitive trips ever. In fact, it is our cognitive abilities that differentiate us from other species, and the ability to plan, organize, fantasize, and evaluate is essential in allowing us to live the type of lives that we may want. However, as this example illustrates, at the times when our thoughts are not our best friend, our mind trips can get us into trouble. Therefore, acting in the moment, with full awareness, is arguably the best effective action to take.

A lack of contact with the present moment can create more than just unpleasant scenarios. Human tendencies to brood and ruminate over past mistakes and failures can elicit feelings of guilt, regret, anxiety, and sadness. Worrying about the future or "future-tripping" can ignite similar emotions. Preoccupation with distressing events, thoughts, and feelings can enhance the distress and contribute to ineffective action or lack of action altogether. When one's life is completely occupied with moments from the past or the future, there is very little room for the present moment. When an effort is made to address the thoughts of the past and future in an effective way change can take place.

If you do not have a history of meditation, staying consistently in the present moment for long periods is exceedingly unrealistic. Humans use language to uncover and process their feelings. With such a long history of linguistic ability, it would not make sense for an acceptance and commitment therapist to encourage a patient to turn off the language and focus on the present moment in silence. That is why the realistic notion in therapy is to teach a patient how to focus on the moment intermittently.[13] This can be achieved by encouraging focus on breathing, while paying attention to distracting thoughts and gently guiding focus back on to the breath. Continually focusing attention on the breath can also be incredibly challenging. Likely, a person can get carried away on a train of thought for a few seconds, as well as being distracted by outside events in the three-minute-breathing period. The reality is such that in our fast-paced world we are constantly expected to pay attention, plan ahead, and remember events to function, be employed, and run a household. Any behavior that teaches one to disengage from thinking, planning, and remembering is counterproductive, unlearned, and comes far and few between. However, not all is lost. With practice, many learn to redirect attention to the present moment, and gain valuable insight as to what the present moment can bring. The more one practices attending to the present moment, the better one can get at disengaging from negative, unhelpful thoughts. Ultimately, the practice of ACT, teaches patients to not consistently be in the present moment, but consistently return to the present moment after being pulled away by distressing thoughts.[14] This act alone can make a difference in how quickly patients can learn ways to manage anxiety, or any type of distress that we are all prone to occasionally.

A large chunk of the work involved in ACT involves values. By definition, a value can be anything that a patient desires as a life outcome. For an acceptance and commitment clinician, values are approached from a behavioral stance where a therapist would encourage ways of behaving that would be consistent with a particular patient's values. For example, if a patient valued family and close intimate relationships, then an acceptance and commitment clinician would work with the patient on helping her behave in such a way that would ultimately increase the likelihood of developing and maintaining close relationships.[15] This philosophy is one that presupposes that although outcomes and consequences are outside the realm of human control, the behavior is something that is within one's locus of control, and one can act in a fashion that can be consistent with achieving the desired goals and results.

ACT specifically highlights valued living as opposed to values alone. At times, behaviors that patients have to engage in to reach the type of value that they desire may be difficult or unpleasant. A woman who specifically values a healthy lifestyle may not always find it easy to find time or energy to engage in exercise or eat healthy foods. Regardless of the challenge, however, ACT states that engaging in valued living is precisely what will reinforce even the undesirable behaviors at the end of the day. Another example is a father who struggles to engage his three-year-old daughter after coming home from work. The father's heartfelt value of being a good parent is in dissonance with his behaviors. Her frequent interruptions during his "wind-down" times are less than desirable. Regardless of the undesirability however, an acceptance and commitment therapist would encourage the father to listen fully and engage with his daughter at the end of the day, and thus reinforce his parenting value. In such manner, when a behavior is fully reinforced, a sense of meaning and purpose for patients is to engage fully in their lives, and participate in activities that were previously unpleasant and cumbersome.[16]

The last piece of ACT is the "commitment" piece. From an ACT perspective, a commitment may imply several things. On the one hand, commitment can mean that one will keep true to one's values and commit to valued living. On the other hand, commitment also involves not engaging in those behaviors inconsistent with one's values. Commitment can also involve engaging in distressing thoughts and emotions of having to exercise the challenging behaviors that might get one closer to one's goal of valued living. For example, a woman who values living a healthy life may go to the gym at the end of a long, hard workday and tolerates the distress of realization that she may not want to go, while fighting fatigue or other factors. Commitment may also involve specifying concrete actions that can be taken to move toward one's goals. Planning, looking ahead, and utilizing strategies are helpful when sizable cognitive and emotional barriers get in the way of valued living. In ACT, commitment is viewed as a moment-by-moment choice exercised daily. Patients who are overwhelmed with having to commit to a certain set of behaviors to achieve a value can be reminded that a never-ending commitment is viewed as a thought. What remains is patients making a choice to live according to the values that they have set up for themselves. On occasion, even the most committed can engage in behaviors not consistent with their values. In such cases, it is common for patients to lose motivation and get discouraged, acting as if all is lost and cannot be gained back. However, the premise of ACT is moment-by-moment living. Therefore, a patient can make a choice in the next moment to live and behave according to one's values. A good analogy for this can be learning how to ice skate and falling down many times before getting up and trying again. From this perspective, patients continue making choices as they live their lives, moment by moment, without feeling the obligatory need to act a certain way for a lifetime, which may seem binding and overwhelming.[17]

What can you expect when walking through the door to sit across from an acceptance and commitment therapist? Well, the initial assessment allows clinicians to understand what patients want from therapy and a big chunk of the conversation is around goal setting as well as life's values. From the onset, an acceptance and commitment therapist engages patients in conversation around the particular avoidance strategies that help them get through their day. The conversations then turn to whether those strategies have helped the patients move toward their goals and the benefits of engaging in the same type of behaviors in the future. The initial assessment stage is explorative and involves the treating clinician engaging the patient in discussions around how past strategies have helped maintain an existing set of issues and what has been done differently to resolve the problems. An example would be an acceptance and commitment therapist asking a patient for a list of strategies that the patient employed in an effort to deal with issues of depression. After generating a list, a therapist might then explore with the patient how effective the strategies have been and whether the behaviors the patient is engaging in currently help move him in the direction of living life according to one's values. A brief glimpse into an ACT session may look something like this:

Therapist: So you are here today to figure out how you might be able to manage your depression better.

Patient: That's the problem. I have been able to do my work in the past, but lately, I have had trouble getting out of the house and even going to work. Most days I call in sick and hope I won't lose my job. I just cannot face anyone anymore and feel like I have lost all hope.

Therapist: Human minds do tend to go into the most darkest of places sometimes. Fortunately you are not alone in this and everyone is prone to negative, unhelpful thoughts every now and then.

Patient: I know that depression runs in my family, but I never thought that it would be this bad for me.

Therapist: Can you give me a recent example of the way depression has been taking control of your life?

Patient: Well, recently I have found myself sitting home alone, dwelling on the negative . . . like I am too stupid to get promoted at work and will never be able to date anyone again, because I am a loser and can barely support myself on the salary that I am currently earning.

Therapist: Right, so your mind is telling you that you may never be able to get out of this hole that you find yourself in and dwelling on this is all you can do to address the issue.

Patient: I guess so. I suppose dwelling on the issue is me trying to get it into some sort of perspective.

Therapist: What do you hope will happen if you continue to dwell and brood over the issue?

Patient: Well, I suppose all I want is some peace and by dwelling, I hope to come to some sort of resolution, so that I am not so sad all the time.

Therapist: And how is this strategy working out for you? Do you find that brooding on the issue is helping you move toward a resolution?

Patient: It actually does help to an extent, until I fall into a deeper hole and have to brood and dwell some more.

Therapist: So dwelling on these issues does help in the short term, but you tend to have to do it over and over again in order to rationalize new material.

Patient: I guess this strategy is not a good long-term strategy and keeps me in my house sad and depressed.

As noted here, an acceptance and commitment therapist will assess the workability of a strategy used and whether a particular strategy ultimately helps move a patient toward valued living. Moreover, evaluation of negative thoughts, emotions, memories, and physical sensations is a constant in ACT work, and a patient is asked to examine whether certain life's values are abandoned or neglected as a result of the presenting concern. Such information is generally elicited through the course of a single session, and discussion with the patient on how his life has changed as a result of presenting issues or symptoms.

During the explorative stage, a therapist would maintain a nonjudgmental and curious attitude, inquiring further into the functionality of a patient's coping strategies and behaviors tried in the past to address an issue. A big piece is understanding how a patient's coping strategy worked for him, and if there is a secondary gain or function that a maladaptive strategy has served. To ensure a nonjudgmental approach, an acceptance and commitment therapist continually encourages the patient to look to his own experience when evaluating results or strategies used. The approach is rooted in validation and assisting the patient in making decisions around choices and strategies to be tested in the future.

ACT is ultimately about helping patients pursue valued-based living. Accordingly, ACT's mindfulness and acceptance practices are not just ends but are the means by which patients will empower themselves and build more vital and meaningful lives. At various points in therapy, ACT clinicians demonstrate to their patients that they understand the living that is rooted in practices that are supportive of values. A part of the journey is also the commitment to pursue those values and, together, patient and therapist explore how to best practice applying mindfulness and acceptance skills to all the barriers that may arise in treatment.

At present, at least thirty randomized controlled trials comparing ACT to other methods of treatment have been conducted and published in peer-reviewed journals. Studies involved looked at ACT versus treatment as usual (TAU) in chronic pain management, psychosis, social anxiety, borderline personality disorder, and substance use.[18] ACT treatment effects on medical issues, such as breast cancer, obesity, and epilepsy have also been studied. In virtually all cases, ACT was found to have better results compared to treatment as usual. Some limitations to the studies involved a small sample of patients and more research remains to be conducted in order to draw more conclusive results. Thus, from patient perspective, ask your therapist about his qualifications around provision of ACT treatment and find out more regarding potential benefits to practicing acceptance and commitment strategies in specific cases of symptom management.

4

ASKING THE "RIGHT" QUESTIONS

Only the wounded healer can truly heal.

—Irvin D. Yalom

One of the most difficult aspects is figuring out how to find a therapist who is just "right." Let me begin this chapter by addressing the various avenues used to find a good therapist in your area. Making the decision to go with the first referral can be nerve-racking, let alone making the appointment and sitting in the waiting room anticipating the therapist's arrival. By the time you walk into your first session, you could be a giddy mess. Taking into account the possible scenarios that could happen if you pick a therapist without doing any outside research, it is important to do what you can to be more comfortable.

When I reflect on my experiences with seeing clients for the first time, many did not know anything about me when first walking through my door. If this has been your experience as well, remember to do the following: research, research, and more research. For convenience sake, I suggest three great websites to check regularly for therapists in your area. First, Psychology Today, www.psychologytoday.com, is a great source for finding the "right" therapist. This website is easy to navigate and has one of the tabs labeled as "Find a therapist." A number of therapists should appear in the window, once you put in your zip code. Take your time and browse through each one, carefully noting each therapist's areas of specialty, and the specific theoretical orientations used. This gives you a good idea as to the type of therapy you will be receiving (i.e., long-term or short-term) as well as whether a particular clinician will be able to address your set of symptoms given their experience and areas of expertise.

Another good site for finding a therapist in your area is the American Psychological Association (APA). The psychologist locator in the APA help center or, www.locator.apa.org, contains several fields that when filled out will give a list of appropriate psychologists in the area given your particular issues. I like the APA site because, unlike Psychology Today, it has a field for the type of problem for which you are seeking help, for example, depression, bipolar disorder, or anxiety. Contrasting the Psychology Today website to the APA site, the APA does not include master's level practitioners in their list of available therapists, which can be a limitation, especially if a number of experienced and well-known master's level clinicians are in the area. Moreover, master's level clinicians usually have as much experience as doctorate level practitioners and may charge a lesser hourly fee for their services. An organization that will provide you with a list of master's level practitioners in your area is the California Association of Marriage and Family Therapists (CAMFT). Other states may have similar resources, which may require a bit of research. Other sites for locating therapists include specialty specific treatment areas, such as the Trichotillomania Learning Center for problems with skin picking or hair pulling. Others include Anxiety and Depression Association of America (ADAA) for various anxiety or depressive disorders, or orientation specific associations such as the Association for Behavioral and Cognitive Therapies. Each site has a tab for locating a therapist in your area and provides some information on latest developments in the field. The last and final method of locating a therapist in the area can be a referral from your general practitioner or a psychiatrist. Generally, a referral from a clinician can be sound, although additional research may be beneficial.

Now you know where to find a therapist, however, a dilemma remains: how to find the right therapist versus the good enough therapist. After browsing several websites, you have narrowed down a therapist that you think is "your guy." You are now ready to pick up the phone and schedule that first appointment. As a clinician myself, I expect the first phone call from clients to be a general description of the presenting problem as well as a discussion around available times, fees, and types of services provided. Unfortunately I rarely have a call from a client who asks me questions about my experience and level of expertise with the presented symptomatology. At the end of the initial phone screening, I make time to ask the client if he has any questions for me. I suspect that this is not the case with most phone consultations. Therefore, it is essential that you take the time to ask the "right" questions before you obligate yourself to a face-to-face appointment.

From my perspective, finding a good enough therapist—a therapist who is caring, empathetic, attuned, and available—is easy. After all, therapists should be good listeners and empathetically respond to their clients. Therapists who are masters in their field, however, are not only expected to have these qualities, but continue to stay current in the latest research for the delivery of best available treatment strategies, and seek out relevant trainings and consultations. These therapists also have their own therapists to work through personal concerns, as well as a way to measure client outcomes and services provided on the regular basis. That is why as a consumer, it is important to ask your potential therapist four basic questions before committing to therapy:

- How do you stay current in the latest research?
- Do you consult on cases with others and, if so, how regularly do you consult?
- Do you receive personal psychotherapy services?
- How do you measure outcomes data and how will our work together be evaluated on the regular basis?

Do not be afraid to lean forward and wrinkle your brow if your therapist does not provide adequate answers to these questions. It is far better to find out if you will be working with the "right" therapist than figure out later that you have spent an exorbitant amount of time and money on someone unable to help you with your initial presenting concerns.

Let's discuss these four questions in more detail to give you a better understanding of why asking these questions is crucial to your success in therapy.

Staying current in the field is a must for any clinician. Therapists are ethically obligated to stay informed of the latest research to deliver best possible treatment. To ensure a successful treatment outcome, clients are encouraged to ask therapists whether they have attended recent conferences, conventions, consultation groups, and other therapeutically relevant venues to ensure access to the latest well-researched treatment methods. The practical implication of this is related to how well a particular clinician can meet a client's need based on his current knowledge and skills. Beyond increasing the overall effectiveness of therapy, several other advantages could be realized with the introduction of a clinician who keeps current. First, having a choice and an understanding of what treatments are available can give consumers a real voice in the type of treatment they choose to receive. This could, in theory, align the therapist and client more closely, focusing on the best available treatment delivery. In my opinion, giving clients a voice in their own care generally contributes to the success of treatment. Over the years, consumers may have grown tired of complacently receiving services that a clinician may offer, and actually want to contribute their own thoughts on the type of care they are receiving. Second, as more and more research accrues, the best-known treatments are continually changing. Once the latest research is available, clinicians should have the knowledge and appropriate skill to implement new tools in treatment. A well-focused therapeutic service should always contain an evaluation of sound research and eliminate the outdated service practices. Admittedly, the pull toward the old and familiar practices is strong for many practicing clinicians in the field. The old models for psychotherapy remain robust; however, for individual practitioners to deliver the best possible services, an implementation of the latest science is required. Therefore, I strongly urge every consumer to ask their therapist about their methods of practice and how they stay current in their field of clinical practice.

Consulting on cases with other practicing clinicians in the field is yet another "must" and a good question to ask your therapist in the initial stages of treatment. This question goes hand in hand with another question, assessing whether your therapist seeks out his own individual therapy. The reason why this is especially crucial to your therapy has to do with management of countertransference on the part of your therapist. Countertransference refers to your therapist's reaction, in which unresolved conflicts may be triggered based on the similarity of unconsciously involved material in the therapist's own life. Quite a bit of research suggests that if left unresolved, countertransference in treatment hinders the progress of psychotherapy. On the other hand, effectively seeking individual therapy and not acting out countertransference aids the therapeutic process and most likely the outcome of therapy.

Over the years of providing psychotherapy to others, I have had issues come up where I have felt jealousy, anger, or guilt over something someone said during the therapeutic encounter. These realizations are humbling and often confusing for therapists. Moreover, clinicians can impede the progress of treatment if these internal struggles are not dealt with in a timely manner. The journey that every mental health professional takes inward at examining his own thoughts is just as important as the ability to be a great therapist. Part of being a wise practitioner in the field is realizing that it is difficult to turn off your own psychological insecurities and difficulties. Striking a balance between self needs and client needs is an important step at providing honest and realistic help to others. Receiving regular consultations and individual help can serve to make your therapist a better one, by eliminating the unnecessary distractions and incorporating self-care as part of the job of being an excellent therapist.

Effective clinicians conduct therapy based on outcomes-informed care. What does that mean? First, every clinician should produce evidence of his clinical effectiveness on a regular basis. Essentially, at the time of each session, your therapist should collect outcomes data to monitor the progress that you are making in therapy. A variety of outcomes data measurement tools are available for therapists to choose, and special software programs make it easy to track psychometric measures. For example, tools are in place to measure a patient's weekly anxiety and depression scores. Once the data are gathered, your therapist can chart your scores over the course of the entire treatment period and together, you can assess whether the levels of anxiety and depression have decreased, increased, or remained the same.

Additionally, your therapist should be educating you about the evidence for outcomes-informed care and the importance of eliciting your feedback at the end of each session. This allows for several factors in the treatment process. First, by initiating both positive and negative feedback therapists can model openness and probably some humility, given that constructive feedback in therapy is not always positive. Ethically, therapists have to always be looking for ways to improve their approach to treatment. Taking advantage of balanced feedback allows therapists to adjust their treatment and work collaboratively with clients to set up the type of intervention care that has the highest success rate. Knowing what works and what does not work in therapy for a particular client represents a reliable and feasible way to deliver consistent successful outcomes.

Purposeful and regular gathering of patient progress is the core element of therapeutic change. It is far better to know whether a therapist is a type of clinician that takes advantage of the latest research and patient feedback than to be stuck in an unproductive weekly cycle with someone who is not current or amenable to patient feedback. What is probably more advantageous for you to understand is that outcomes-informed care places a measure of accountability on the therapist. Weekly monitoring as well as feedback provides proof of value and evidence of return on the investment (psychotherapeutic process). Using client feedback on the regular basis is by far the strongest recommendation to come from this book. If your therapist is not regularly checking in with you and monitoring your progress, then it is probably time to find yourself another therapist. As stated previously, the tools available to measure outcomes data are many, and your therapist should be taking advantage of outcomes-informed care.

Understanding how to choose the "right" therapist can be challenging. Asking mental health professionals tough questions in the beginning can go a long way toward bringing you satisfaction in psychotherapy. Making sure that your therapist stays current, knowledgeable, and accountable for the services she provides is a smart approach to receiving the best possible care. Far gone are the days when just building a relationship with clients and talking about a particular therapeutic approach used are enough. Therapists really should be concerned with showing how their treatment can yield positive results and demonstrating current knowledge in the field. The "right" therapist translates into the type of treatment that "works" for the client, and the money paid is "well spent." Asking your therapist questions should be second nature to all prospective clients, as this way assesses whether a particular psychotherapeutic practice is successful. Just as with any business, therapists begin their practice with clients and concentrate on their needs.

I will close out this chapter by mentioning that there has been a recent, significant shift in the field of psychotherapy. The latest research suggests that placing an emphasis on gathering outcomes data as well as encouraging client feedback, corresponds to the level of success and improvement in therapy. The two factors alone yield the most impressive and clinically significant change in treatment outcomes. In fact, client deterioration scores are cut in half, along with dropout rates, if outcomes measures are in place.[1] Feedback and regular monitoring allows therapists to tailor individual treatment on the regular basis, taking into account client response to specific interventions and client preference in the choice of interventions used. In short, asking the right questions could make a difference between the "right" and the "good enough" therapist.

5

THE VULNERABLE PATIENT

The best years of your life are the ones in which you decide your problems are your own. You do not blame them on your mother, the ecology, or the president. You realize that you control your own destiny.

—Albert Ellis

I suppose there is no easy way to tell people that you may have a mental illness or require services from a mental health professional. Often, even making the decision to go to a therapist can be a torturous one. Despite the fact that people today seek out therapeutic services, many still show up to my first appointment deeply troubled at having to be in therapy. The thought of discussing their most intimate feelings or touching upon the problems that brought them to therapy is inconceivable. Much of this reluctance most likely is for personal and professional reasons, but it is also from jokes, cruelty, or poor reactions from colleagues, friends, or relatives. Reluctance to attend therapy can also be a result of cultural reasons, such as a general belief that personal issues have to stay personal. Clients are often concerned with what other people will think of them or even if they will be viewed differently as a result of being in therapy.

Unfortunately still today quite a bit of stigma is attached to mental illness. There is however, a slow growing realization in our culture that a positive sense has to develop in regards to seeking out therapeutic services to establish a healthy personal and group identity. At the same time, many continue to shy away from psychotherapy and turn to other methods when needing help. When the option of psychotherapy is erased due to stigma, many turn to self-help groups, yoga, crystals, special food remedies, religion, and chiropractors to target their symptoms. There are a number of factors that influence the decision-making process for people. And yet still, when individuals decide to deal with their illnesses in a different manner from what is accepted by the dominant culture, they are labeled as "crazy," "weird," or "abnormal." What are the options available for people? If talking to a professional is not accepted and exploring other methods is viewed as strange, what should one consider as an acceptable form of help?

On average, people are more likely to avoid psychotherapeutic services due to negative family attitudes and specific negative beliefs around treatment. Some common factors include not wanting to appear weak for needing psychological assistance, family biases, and negative cultural implications. Therefore it is unfortunate that other people's perceptions and negative identification with counseling services can and do hinder people from getting the needed help. This of course makes the lives of those who could benefit from "talk therapy" unnecessarily more difficult. This chapter illustrates that stigma is a complex phenomenon that has a broad and harmful effect on those suffering with mental illness. As you read the next several pages, use this information to help yourselves and people with mental illness better deal with stigma.

Due to stigma around mental health services, it is hard nowadays to find a patient who does not feel a certain measure of discomfort to being in therapy. Therefore, to treat any type of mental health issue without taking into account a measure of stigma attached to being in counseling is equally hard. However, a number of recent changes have helped those in treatment to deal with the effects of stigmatization. In addition to treating the primary presenting symptoms, clinicians in the area of cognitive therapy have also begun to understand stigma from unhelpful self-statements or cognitions that are played out in people's heads, much like broken song tracks. These cognitive self-statements have developed as a result of socialization in our culture. These self-statements may explain the reason behind why some people overcome the effects of stigma and seek out therapeutic services, and others continue to be unmotivated into action because of it. What are some ways for patients to deal with the effects of stigma of being in treatment?

Cognitive therapy has shown results in helping people change their cognitions that lead to anxiety, depression, and self-stigma about being in therapy. Clinicians assist clients in reframing their unhelpful and distressing thoughts by targeting their belief systems around stigma, reviewing the evidence, and assessing the emotional costs of spending time and effort interpreting thoughts and actions of others. Several published research trials have found that these types of interventions have resulted in a significant reduction of symptoms around self-stigma and suggest that the types of cognitive interventions used are not only helpful, but also necessary in the treatment process.[1]

Another powerful intervention approach to changing unhelpful self-talk is personal empowerment. As a rule, people feel empowered when they have a measure of control over their own lives and their treatment process. People who feel empowered are expected to have high self-efficacy and high self-esteem. These individuals are not bogged down by labels, stigma, and their own symptomatology, but have a good outlook and take an active, knowledgeable role in their own recovery. That is why it is imperative that therapists foster personal empowerment among clients by giving them a choice and greater control over their treatment process. This involves a collaborative form of planning, in which the client takes an active role in the development of the treatment versus passively relying on the therapist's knowledge to pave a way to recovery.

Beyond the tools of empowerment and cognitive therapy, yet another way to overcome self-stigma is reaching certain goals in therapy, beyond mental health. The ability of clients to use self-determination to achieve success in areas of employment, academics, finances, housing, and other aspects of social life can be a powerful intervention in therapy for overcoming stigmatization. Rather than isolating and shying away from communities, clients in therapy can continue making efforts to adapt to community living despite negative labels for being in therapy. Encouraging clients to set goals in treatment that promote community integration can prepare clients for independent social functioning.

Consumers of "talk therapy" can also empower themselves by becoming involved in efforts to recognize and fight stigma around mental illness. Clients can organize walks and rallies that acknowledge most people's struggle with mental illness and create their own avenues for destigmatization. By involving themselves in community efforts, clients focus on their strengths rather than weaknesses, and continue to further promote social awareness and integration. It is important to note however, that the effort of destigmatization involves more than one individual. Society level interventions are more powerful when dealing with stereotypes, discrimination, and prejudice than individual level change. With that in mind, although stigma cannot be considered as an individual problem, individual-level interventions are still useful and efficacious when working with clients. To that extent, this type of perspective may help individuals understand the ways to overcome stigma around seeking mental health help. Clients can also learn how to deal with the threat of stigma for themselves and focus on other issues relevant to mental health and well-being.

It may be beneficial to devote a bit of time to additionally explore the cost and benefit analysis of disclosing one's experience with mental illness. I will preface this section by stating that all readers of this book should consider their personal perceptions of the costs and benefits behind disclosure. Perhaps the harshest and most sobering consequence of disclosure around mental illness is the amount of hate crimes regularly reported on nightly news. The sheer amount of violence would make anyone think twice before openly discussing their particular mental health issues with anyone, including their own family members. Other examples exist, ones that are less harsh, but nonetheless are still hurtful, such as experiencing disapproval from others, as well as general avoidance of people who are perceived to be "in treatment for mental concerns." This kind of stress experienced on a regular basis results in low self-esteem by those contemplating treatment. Research suggests that the stress has the potential to drive many teens and adults to suicide as well as a variety of other consequences (drugs, prostitution, and other dangerous or violent behaviors).[2] Based on these disadvantages alone, I would be concerned with telling any patient to disclose his mental status. On the other hand, research has clearly demonstrated that there are benefits to disclosing one's struggles with mental health issues. The largest, and perhaps the most important advantage of disclosure, is no longer having to keep a secret. The alleviation of stress alone is enough to qualify this as an advantage. Disclosing struggles with mental health results in the ability to build better interpersonal relationships and allows for a possibility of support from families and loved ones. Another potential benefit of disclosure can serve the function of a warning for someone who is predisposed to certain mental illness within the family. Learning more about a particular mental disorder early on can prevent someone from engaging in certain dangerous behaviors, such as the use and abuse of alcohol or other substances. Substance abuse has been linked to exacerbation of symptoms of many mental disorders and has been demonstrated in studies to considerably impair the outcome of recovery.[3] Unfortunately, there is no clear formula for how things will shake out when an individual chooses to admit and reveal the presence of mental illness. Therefore, it is the responsibility of the individual alone to consider all the advantages and disadvantages inherent in disclosure.

In an effort to fight stigma, many antistigma campaigns use education as a valuable approach to teaching others about mental illness. Unfortunately, in spite of good intentions, these campaigns often focus on the biological explanations of mental illness, which has been found to be unhelpful among cultures. By framing mental illness as a biological disease, other people receive the message that those struggling with mental illness are helpless and have to be taken care of by others. Although the intention of these campaigns is well meaning, the result is often disempowering. Biological explanations may imply that people suffering with mental illness have no control over their behaviors, are unpredictable, and may be even violent. In contrast, much research has been devoted to promoting another type of education, an education that focuses on the psychosocial explanations behind mental illness. Instead of underlining the cellular mechanisms responsible for mental illness, psychosocial explanations rely on understanding mental disorders through an environmental and trauma perspective. These types of explanations take into account poverty, childhood abuse, and lack of a social support system as an undercurrent for mental illness. The idea behind this type of psychoeducation is to reframe psychiatric symptoms as understandable reactions to life's stressors. Studies focusing on changing negative beliefs associated with mental illness have found psychosocial explanations to be more effective at improving attitudes and lifting negative beliefs associated with stigma around mental illness.[4]

In recent years, in the United States alone, many antistigma campaigns were held with the goal of improving attitudes about mental illness. Many organizations are jumping in to fight the fight of stigma. However, as discussed earlier in this chapter, efforts have to be made to research more carefully the type of campaign messages that are most effective at winning this fight. For starters, learning more about the perceived attitudes to certain types of content, medium, and strategy is important to distributing the type of message that leads to implementation of positive changes. This is an important point to consider, as the image resulting from stigmatization of people with mental illness cannot necessarily be separated from the available mental health treatment itself. If the general attitude about people with mental illness is negative, the profession of mental health counseling will implicitly suffer the same fate, and the public is in danger of questioning the efficacy and credibility of psychotherapeutic work. On the other hand, establishing and delivering an antistigma campaign that works can brand psychotherapy as a symbol of health, prevention, and hope, thereby popularizing mental health services and reducing stigma.

If I had to state my thoughts on our, as a society, possible success at combating stigma in the next few decades, the phrase I would use would be "restrained optimism." Am I so naïve as to forget thousands of years of human history, cross-cultural differences, and the hard-wired tendencies of all humans to ostracize and stigmatize certain groups? The answer is of course "no." However, it is possible to conceive of an idea, that there might be another push in human history where we could triumph over ignorance and embrace our inner compassion. With the advance of technology and education, I am swayed to believe that humans could emphasize justice and equality and overcome their prejudices. I am inclined to point out that this effort will take a long, well-researched, and dedicated approach. This effort will involve changes in the media, workforce, and communities to encourage people suffering with mental illness to seek out adequate treatment. Moreover, it will take creative and new ways at educating people about mental illness and perhaps even exposing individuals to the personal and family struggles of living with daily realities of mental illness. Over my years of practicing, I still retain the belief that for many, mental illness holds the aura of mystery, confusion, and danger. Perhaps advertising stories of courage, compassion, and resilience can be incorporated into every antistigma campaign for the general public to understand the true nature of the beast. Stories on individual successes in treatment rarely make the nightly news, and instead, television screens in every house portray tales of horror, danger, loss, and helplessness. Perhaps in the next few years, people will begin to understand that we cannot afford to bury realities, and for every gruesome portrayal of mental illness, a related success is comparable to sensational headlines. The challenge is here and very real. Changes are necessary, and we all can stand to benefit from joining this particular fight.

6

BEHIND PSYCHIATRIC DRUGS

However beautiful the strategy, you should occasionally look at the results.

—Winston Churchill

The Agency for Healthcare Research and Quality reports that in the United States alone, the number of people using psychiatric drugs has increased from 21 million in 1997 to 32.6 million in 2004.[1] The astronomical figures lead to the conclusion that psychiatric drugs are the first line of defense in battling mental illness, with behavioral and cognitive interventions remaining on the decline. Today, treatment for mental illness means medication. But what does it mean for clinically supported research trials? In this chapter I address the subject of risks and benefits behind major psychiatric drugs, providing a reference for readers to evaluate and examine current drug literature to facilitate medication decisions.

I begin with a discussion of antidepressant medications, which account for the greatest expenditure of all the psychotropic drugs in the treatment of mental illness.[2] Typically, antidepressants are the common treatment for mild to moderate depression and are stated to be effective and safe, causing only minor, temporary side effects. Examining the empirical research, however, paints a different picture altogether. In the review of all the studies that have looked at the efficacy of antidepressants, research has found that the claim that antidepressants actually help with depression is inconsistent. In fact, empirical evidence suggests that those on antidepressant medication experience longer depressive episodes, and the number of episodes is actually higher for nonusers. This proposes that the general assumption behind the efficacy of antidepressants needs to be examined further, and the emerging research is inconsistent with the prevalent assumptions. Moreover, a meta-analytical review examining the success rate of antidepressant medications has found that nearly 82 percent of results was duplicated by placebo control groups. Adding to the critique, examination of all trials submitted to the Food and Drug Administration (FDA) for popular antidepressants found no clinical benefit between the antidepressant group and placebo, with the exception of the most severely depressed group.

Recently, a great deal of focus has been on the assumption that concurrent psychopharmacological and psychotherapeutic treatment can alleviate depression better versus any one treatment alone. Unfortunately, once again, empirical evidence demonstrates that there is no advantage to combining the two treatments for better outcomes. Thase and colleagues report that combining two treatments does offer some benefit to individuals suffering with recurrent, severe depression after twelve weeks of treatment; however, this outcome is not observed in cases of mild depression.[3] Given these findings, readers should proceed with caution and beware of the risks and benefits of taking antidepressants. The negligible benefits of selective serotonin reuptake inhibitors (SSRIs) over placebo highlight the importance of weighing out the risks of taking this particular class of drugs. Common side effects are: agitation, sleep disturbance, and gastrointestinal and sexual complications. Another factor are possible drug-drug interactions if taking more than just antidepressants. Always review the evidence for efficacy and safety of any major drug classes for all age groups.

The second major classification of drugs is antipsychotics. Much like antidepressants, antipsychotics have made their appearance in mental healthcare settings beyond just hospitals and clinics. Many diagnosed with bipolar disorder and other nonpsychotic problems are prescribed antipsychotic medications and, in fact, prescription rates for antipsychotics tripled between 1998 and 2002.[4] For those suffering with psychotic disorders such as schizophrenia, antipsychotic medication is a requirement for management of severe symptoms associated with the disorder. The diagnosis is often viewed as "untreatable" and requires a constant regimen of medication. But what about those who are not diagnosed with a disorder manifesting psychotic symptoms? Is there evidence for recovery that does not entail a regular drug regimen and, if so, why are antipsychotics still being prescribed?

Results from several trials funded by the National Institute of Mental Health (NIMH) confirm that many patients report antipsychotic medication does not improve their general quality of life. In fact, many are burdened by the side effects of the medication overall and discontinue use after eighteen months. Many patients suffering with psychotic disorders find that the side effects of antipsychotic medication outweigh the benefits and struggle to tolerate use for an extended period. For those who do continue taking antipsychotics, remission from clinically defined symptoms still does not help with social functioning and integration, with patients continuing to struggle with issues of isolation and loneliness.[5]

Similarly, prescription for children does not stop with antidepressants or stimulants. Medical prescribers are increasingly favoring the use of antipsychotics and hypertensives to treat diagnoses of bipolar disorder in all children. A study by Moreno and colleagues has found a steady increase in the diagnosis of bipolar disorder among children between the ages of one to nineteen years. Of the children diagnosed with the disorder, 90 percent were treated with psychoactive drugs, half of which were antipsychotic in nature. Most of the children investigated in the study were receiving more than one drug and only four out of ten received any type of psychotherapeutic services along with their prescribed medications.[6] Interestingly enough, antipsychotic medication is also beginning to be widely used in the treatment of ADHD among children. These psychoactive drugs are favored in the management of ADHD symptoms such as aggression, irritability, and other conduct-related behaviors.[7] The two most popular diagnoses among kids today are bipolar disorder and ADHD, accounting for about 50 percent of all the antipsychotics used in this sample population.[8]

Perhaps the most disturbing news comes in the form of a group put together by the APA. Results support the finding that most studies promoting use of antipsychotic medications to treat children have a number of eye-opening limitations. These limitations include a small sample size of subjects enrolled in studies, open trials in which the participants and researchers know which treatment is being administered thereby maximizing the potential for bias, as well as analysis of data with a retrospective review, which has been largely unrecognized in child and adolescent psychiatry. Nevertheless, with industry-funded research, the FDA continues to issue approval for drugs with poor study design and scope. Unfortunately, aside from the poor study design, the number and magnitude of side effects are also underreported, and the evidence is constructed in such a way as to minimize the potential for doubt in use of many antipsychotic medications. In an NIMH-funded study comparing several antipsychotics, the primary outcome measure was not clinical improvement or remission of symptoms, but discontinuation from the treatment. The study design made it possible to evaluate the results in such a way as to foster confidence in the efficacy of the drugs, versus an indication of a poor benchmark for success. The researchers and participants did not know of the drugs they were taking, thus making the sites triple blind; however, there was no placebo group, flexible dosage administration, and little by way of an exclusion criteria for multiple additional drugs in use by the study participants. The goal of the study was an evaluation of how each antipsychotic medication tested compared with the other, under clinical conditions, as well as real-world response rates. Results from the study confirmed that many patients were burdened by the number of side effects from the drugs and many discontinued before the end of the study. Thus, systematic treatment of patients using antipsychotic medications has to be examined further. The claims of superiority of these drugs are often largely exaggerated, perhaps inspired by patient desperation, as well as clinical need for truly effective agents to treat severe mental illness. Another factor to note in the success of medication with little evidential support is the aggressive marketing techniques of these drugs. This allows the public to enhance the perception of the effectiveness of medication in absence of solid empirical research. Of note, remission of symptoms for any agent on the market does not merit adequate social or cognitive functioning for those suffering with disorders entailing use of antipsychotics, and this highlights the need for psychosocial interventions.

Given some of the dangers inherent in the use of psychotropic medications, it would be worthwhile to discuss the critical flaws inherent in for-profit industries that play a role in fashioning all the new drugs.

Sadly, the federally governed agencies and academic advisory boards are not the health guards that they are expected to be. Actually, in a Pulitzer Prize report, Willman investigated the far-reaching ties that the National Institutes of Health (NIH) and the FDA had to pharmaceutical companies. In the report, Willman discussed the strong affiliation between those that develop and modify the diagnostic criteria behind mental illness and those that spend their time and money developing new psychotropic agents to target the symptoms of the diagnoses found in the *Diagnostic and Statistical Manual of Mental Disorders*.[9] Reading Willman's report, it seems unlikely that there exists today good and pure investigative science that does not rely on industry money for its source of materials and study design. The result is a direct correlation between those who fund the studies and their outcomes.

In considering psychotropic agents, many psychiatric drug studies tend to minimize and underreport adverse drug reactions. As a result, many side effects are not assessed properly and may not even appear on the label.[10] Clinical publications typically discuss adverse drug effects in the discussion section of papers, highlighting the limitations in a narrative format. Presenting data in such a way allows the authors to assert that drugs are safe, when in fact if the data had been presented in a statistically significant format with tables and comparison charts, it would have been easy to see that safety concerns are not reported at all.

Additionally, when psychiatric drugs are prescribed, they are generally prescribed to be taken for an extended period. For any medication to integrate and take effect within the body, it may take as long as two or three weeks. There is a conflict again then, when most clinical trials last anywhere from six to twelve weeks and are not measuring drug effectiveness in real-life settings. Without longer terms to follow up, it is difficult to determine the efficacy of any drug on the market. Authors of short-term clinical trials often fail to identify this limitation in the discussion section of the paper, and rush to make conclusions regarding the safety of the tested medication. Thus, time is a consideration when assessing conclusions around superiority of the investigative agent on the basis of a limited trial.

Currently, a huge conflict of interest exists regarding industry influence to report and find only favorable results of the drugs studied. The strategies involved may be comparing the drugs against other less effective drugs, comparing drugs to low doses of existent, popular drugs to prove efficacy, or even comparing drugs to high doses of competitor drugs to show toxicity of other drugs. Overall, study design, data outcomes, and analysis are part of a bigger scheme to push new drugs out into the market without much regard for ethical standards. Knowing these facts is essential when evaluating any clinical drug trial study for a possible consideration of a psychotropic medication in the treatment process. Readers of this book can and should approach any study with a healthy measure of skepticism before drawing any conclusions on the safety and efficacy of a drug. As a point of consideration, knowing that there might be a conflict of interest between pure, investigative science and industry-driven results is essential for evaluating meaningful conclusions of any research. Most well-known academic journals guard readers against this boundary and encourage finding sources and author affiliations before buying into study results. An online database published by a nonprofit group documents researcher conflicts as it touches on studies conducted without disclosure: www.cspinet.org/integrity/.

In discussing the risks inherent in clinical research when it comes to psychotropic medication, always note the benefits of psychiatric drugs. As research and practice have shown, some psychiatric drugs clearly help some adults get better in daily life functioning. Pharmacotherapy also helps some children and adolescents. With that in mind, it is always wise to weigh out the risks and benefits of certain types of drugs. Another option available, aside from pharmacotherapy, involves psychosocial treatments that are grounded in strong evidence-based practices with virtually no adverse effects. For most disorders, there are standalone treatments that work well with symptom management. These treatments are well researched and are indicated to be safer than psychoactive medications. Therefore, in my firm opinion, before children, adolescents, or adults are placed on psychoactive medication, psychosocial treatments in the form of therapy should be explored first. An almost automatic prescription of psychoactive drugs has become so common nowadays that often patients forget to consider other forms of available treatment. Other treatment options do exist however, and patients and practitioners alike should examine the scientific evidence before jumping to medication.

Several conclusions emerge from this chapter. First, readers are encouraged to examine every clinical drug study with a magnifying glass and consider possible clinical implications of the authors' affiliations and study outcomes. The second point to consider is that psychiatric drug treatments should not be the first line of treatment over psychosocial options. These conclusions, however, do not negate the potentially powerful and beneficial effect of certain psychotropic medications, particularly when clients believe that the root cause of their problems is biological in nature and maintain the view that drugs might be helpful. The subject that has not gotten a lot of attention is the efficacy of psychotherapy, which has been supported through evidenced-based research in the domain of symptom distress. Keeping in mind that no scientific justification exists to necessarily use medication first, patients can consider other options available in the treatment process. Researching treatments and making informed decisions will help many choose the type of treatment that fits best with their particular set of values and preferences.

From another angle, a reasonable expectation to have is that a clinician who provides psychotherapeutic services will ultimately introduce the subject of the inherent risks and benefits of any treatment process. A good clinician will never be afraid to discuss the benefits and limitations of all available treatments and even mention personal opinion of the type of treatment they themselves are providing. The treating clinician is responsible for providing families with current information in regards to any treatment option. Similarly, it can be considered an ethical imperative that treatment providers discuss existent conflicts of interest inherent in many medication options, depending on the setting of the prescribing psychiatrist. Risk-benefit discussions are not only necessary, but are the ethical standard in mental health treatment.

In the interest of giving readers some guidelines when choosing a psychotropic medication to better deal with symptoms of a given disorder, here are some steps to help you make an informed decision.

- When initially considering medication, involve as many qualified individuals in your life as you can to help you understand the nature of your condition and the corresponding symptoms.
- Develop an understanding of your mental health illness with respect to not only biological/hereditary causes, but also taking into account environmental, interactional, and sociocultural factors.
- Engage your support network (psychiatrist, mental health clinician, family, friends) in helping you develop a plan to deal with

the distressing psychological symptoms by taking into account your strengths, weaknesses, cultural context, and other preferences.

- When considering medication, make sure all potential benefits, risks, and adverse reactions are understood. Review studies supporting the risks and benefits of the medication and obtain additional sources of information if the reviewed studies are biased.
- Make sure to not sign up for a fixed treatment plan. The treatment process varies from day to day, carefully taking into account a patient's progress and feedback. A treatment plan is something that is always subject to modification depending on the results of treatment. Moreover, a discussion involving medication use and/ or discontinuation is something that has to be part of the treatment process as well, carefully considering the length of treatment and patient response to medication.

In today's society, a prevalent belief is the notion that any medical or mental condition can be targeted through medication treatment. This is unfortunate, given that science clearly indicates that psychological and social processes are the catalysts for change in the biological underwritings of human beings. Although some patients may be helped some of the time with medication, chemical agents may be misdirecting us from understanding the more real and sustainable agents involved in long-term recovery. In the conclusion of this chapter, I really urge the readers to adopt a critical perspective when deciding on a particular mode of treatment, and if possible do the research involved in understanding the potentially dangerous side effects of prescriptive treatment options.

7

INDIVIDUAL VERSUS GROUP THERAPY

If you are going through hell, keep going!

—Winston Churchill

I am frequently asked whether group therapy is an acceptable form of treatment for those who cannot necessarily afford individual therapy. The answer is yes and again yes! Imagine this scene: eight to ten people in a room—strangers—asked to relate, support, share, and listen to one another. Could anything be more challenging and more rewarding? Having led inpatient and outpatient process groups, I have seen results within a single session, where men and women of all walks of life, with a number of varying diagnoses, are thrown together wanting to connect, resolve issues, and matter to another individual in the room. Experiencing similar feelings with different situational circumstances, patients tell their stories uncovering deep roots for everyday problems.

Despite the evident benefits of group therapy, many clinical settings today tend to shy away from providing therapy groups and question their efficacy. The settings that have used group processes to facilitate patient recovery have found them to be incredibly useful. More and more patients are aware of the availability of groups in communities and medical settings and seek to become members. The popular groups would likely include Alcoholics Anonymous, Narcotics Anonymous, Adult Children of Alcoholics, Nicotine Anonymous, Overeaters Anonymous, Sex and Love Addicts Anonymous, and many other twelve-step groups. One particularly important piece of evidence to support the efficacy of group therapy came from studies examining patient recovery outcomes based on short versus long-term hospital stay. To researchers' dismay, the correlate to better patient recovery had to do with the use of more inpatient therapy groups in short-term hospital stays as opposed to longer-term stays. What was even more surprising is that patients who did participate in inpatient therapy groups during their hospitalization were more likely to seek out outpatient therapy groups and continue work on their individual recovery.[1]

Often, to adapt to the harsh realities of life, people seek ingenious ways to avoid the pain and escape reality. These realities may include abusive homes, inability to gain employment or education, financial struggles, or mental illness coupled with substance abuse disorders. Patients find that by attenuating their anxieties in a group therapy setting, they are exposing themselves to their worst fears in the company of peers willing to listen and working through their own anxieties and struggles with life. Group therapy programs are intended to be sensitive to specific needs of specific types of patients, and research does indicate that overall group therapy is even more effective than individual therapy.[2] Group psychotherapy can be for better or worse: if led well, it can be a source of considerable therapeutic benefit.

Therapy groups address several important aspects of the human condition in two ways. First, therapy groups are a small piece of the arena that can hold patients' maladaptive relational patterns that are displayed outside of the group. The group provides a structure, where patients are asked to relate and absorb each other's experiences and understand how certain behavioral patterns that are displayed in the group can affect a certain patient outside of the group when he interacts with family members, friends, or authority figures. The group dynamic helps each member look at specific ongoing patterns in thought as well as behavior that can affect a particular member's relationship with the outside world. Members offer input and use each other for support and feedback. The other aspect of a therapy group that promotes recovery has to do with the ability of patients to relate to one another during the group. A significant amount of data suggests that a patient's ability to relate to others in the group is a big factor in the recovery and outcome process.[3] The group's ability to listen, support, offer constructive feedback, and promote a safe environment for each member can help break down interpersonal barriers. Not only can each member address his own issues within the group, but patients can project their fears onto others (i.e., trust, loyalty, rejection) and attempt to understand why certain members within the group can trigger those feelings. For example, if a member in a group sets out to deal with issues of trust, that member can pick out one or two people in a group that trigger those same feelings of mistrust and identify, with group help, what it is about their behaviors and the interpretation of those behaviors that continues to spin the cycle of mistrust of certain others. Not only is a group setting a great way to address a patient's pressing interpersonal needs, but this is also a form of practice for patients to learn and apply new behaviors when interacting with others in their lives.

Common doubts and fears appear for patients when participating in a group process. Certain questions arise: "Will I be able to speak up in front of a group of people about my problems?" "How much will I really benefit from sharing my issues with a group of strangers?" "Can I trust each member of the group to hold confidentiality of the material I am divulging?" Fortunately, these fears are quickly dispelled in a group with the introduction of group rules as well as a thorough discussion around confidentiality. The group process, with its safe, supportive, mobilizing spirit very rapidly engages each member and alleviates most fears. There are, however, times when select members hesitate to participate in the group and are troubled by even thinking about sharing their intimate life details with strangers. In such cases, the patient should reevaluate participation in a group and consider individual therapy.

I find it beneficial to discuss the process of entrusting others with intimate life secrets in a group setting. After all, this can be a deterrent to enter treatment in a group. Part of human nature is to share and connect with others by consciously or unconsciously divulging content. Even with the best of intentions, some people still find themselves discussing material that belongs to another. Breaking trust and confidentiality is one of the most serious considerations for a group. How then does a group leader handle this process? In practice, fortunately, confidentiality is rarely broken in a group, and most likely has to do with two important factors. When engaging members in a discussion around confidentiality, group leaders encourage participants to use censorship and precaution. If a patient in a group does find himself needing to share interesting details with someone outside of the group, the leaders suggest that this member does not use any specifying data to reveal the identity of another member in a group. This caveat precludes members from breaking confidentiality. Again, possible disclosure by a member with or without identifying information may still be injurious to another member in a group. Generally, such disclosures occur rarely based on another important consideration—dismissal from the group. Members of a group fear group retaliation and even dismissal from therapy. Banishment from a group can be considered one of man's ultimate fears. This innate instinct to belong arguably precludes members from gossiping on the outside or with one another and promotes confidentiality. Yet another important consideration to note is that participants rarely jump into sharing personal, intimate details without first testing the safety of the group. Generally a group would spend time developing safety, trust, and solidarity before leaping into the actual therapy process. Invariably, although this progression may take three to four sessions, it proves to be beneficial for a number of reasons and to all members of a group.

Another question that often comes up in groups is "How can one therapist attend to ten or more members in a one-hour period?" The question is a relatively simple one to answer—this cannot be done. This is the major underlying difference between group and individual therapy processes. One therapist cannot attend to every single member need in a one-hour session, nor is this the goal of group therapy. Rather, the goal of group therapy is to engage members in an interrelational process. A group leader manages multiple interactions involving three, four, or possibly five members, delicately navigating between meaning and process for those members. At that time, the leader is directly involved in pointing out similarities, differences, and conveying the meaning of the relational process to the members directly involved. In a way, a leader has to be intuitive enough to grasp the dynamics of this relational process fairly quickly and figure out how the specific dynamics can be interwoven into the whole pattern of the group.[4] A group leader may even encourage other members to participate in the group interaction who perhaps could relate to the discussion. To draw an analogy to describe the role of a therapist in a group process is perhaps a bit like driving a car. You are paying attention to your own driving while concurrently taking into account everyone else on the road.

Some of you may still wonder about the possible benefit of group therapy with a multitasking leader and little individual one-on-one interaction. What is the advantage of being in therapy with so minimal deserved attention from the leader? One of the benefits is of course that the group therapy modality has the ability to engage those members who would otherwise never consider individual forms of therapy. Additionally, those members who have gone through individual therapy could have perhaps developed negative associations with therapy or found it to be unhelpful overall. Another factor for using group modality is to consider that the group method of treatment can often accelerate recovery for many. For example, a member with a diagnosis of antisocial personality disorder whose ability to form and sustain relationships with others has been impaired, might find group cohesion a unique experience. Developing such an understanding in individual therapy could be beyond clinical capability, whereas a group can engulf members in the growing feeling of togetherness and community belonging that would otherwise be impossible to simulate on the outside. While it is important to mention the opportunities for people to do individual work at one time or another inside the group, the focus cannot be on one specific member for the entirety of group time. The goal is to engage all participants in the group process and develop a broad viewpoint that is the product of participation of everyone in the group.

Individual therapy between two individuals in private can be described as a moment-by-moment reality. But how did it start and why do human beings engage in individual therapy? Most of the literature that you read, no doubt, gives the immediate impression that psychotherapy originated with Freud and did not exist much before him. However, clearly, humans have had emotional, psychological, and spiritual needs for centuries before Freud and will continue to have them for centuries after. Most would agree that early humans fought for food supply, health, predatory threats, in-group conflicts, and other competitive forces. Arguably, human suffering began with small communities of hunters and gatherers, dominating for the right to survive. Even religious accounts describe human beings as losing contact with faith, spirituality, and needing guidance and help. Whether patients present to therapy to establish a connection with another or to work through some internal problem is really a moot point. Thousands of years of existence demonstrated that humans do thrive on emotional connection and intelligence. Many would point out that being human means that we come with a certain set of predetermined characteristics such as aggression, greed, negative thinking, jealousy, etc., that preclude us from functioning successfully with others. Also our nature is to be caring, compassionate, kind, and loving. When certain unhelpful characteristics outweigh the helpful ones is when we find ourselves in the thralls of psychological problems. Also insufficiencies in care, shame, guilt, loss, and abuse explain much of human suffering. While some may argue that we have come far in our advances of medicine, technology, and longevity, and that we now live in a postemotional world, others are very much conflicted and fearful over the loss of humanness that possibly lies beneath all healthy human psychological functioning.

The field of therapy has been created through our psychological distresses and needs. Although the *Diagnostic and Statistical Manual of Mental Disorders* may list only around 350 psychological disorders, a case can be made for psychological distress due to losses, stress, aging, marital discord, and divorce as well as other issues such as irritability, worry, fatigue, and sleep problems. Psychological distress can also be defined in terms of financial distress and physical illness. These diagnostic labels may be somewhat crude, but they give us some idea as to the scope of possible mental health concerns. The implication of psychological distress is clear and points to a necessity to continue to provide quality mental health care. Unfortunately, this need is not always self-evident, and neither is it scientifically justifiable nor universally palatable. The validity of the therapeutic process is often questioned based on insufficient evidence to claim that it works. If we were to look at the academic circles, psychotherapy has always been questioned as a "hard" science as compared to its counterweights such as traditional science and social science. Simultaneously, however, certain encouraging trends have been emerging lately, highlighting the growth and acceptance of psychological counseling and psychotherapy. Growth of demand from the public necessitated the accompanying demand for evidence-based practices in psychotherapy. The emergence of brief models of psychotherapy such as CBT as the treatment of choice with a significant body of research and literature to support its efficacy could seriously threaten the status of psychotherapy as "erroneous and ineffective."

The early dominance of psychoanalytical models has given way to other forms of psychological therapy. This diversification is mainly due to our growth and adaptation of "therapy" to other practices, such as spirituality, psychopharmaceuticals, genetics, and multiculturalism. These trends prompted more research in the fields of neuroscience, biology, and technology, all expanding the standard psychoanalytical practices and individualizing therapeutic treatments to include cognitive, dialectical, and behavioral models. These brief, evidence-based models help the unemployed regain confidence in the job market, the depressed and anxious to use cognitive restructuring to help alleviate and replace unhelpful, automatic thoughts, the bipolar manic to confront uncomfortable feelings and unhelpful behaviors, and the socially isolated to begin learning depersonalization techniques. The field of psychology is growing and becoming more refined in its ways of providing mental health coverage, and the curative process for the patient is becoming more and more concrete. Emphasis is placed on measurable results versus vague lengthy process to self-actualization. History has proven that people invariably inspire change, and I believe the field of psychotherapy has changed radically in the last sixty years, no longer leaving question marks in the minds of many as to whether or not it works.

To the best of my knowledge most folks are familiar with the process of individual therapy. Many patients in individual therapy have learned that it can be a meaningful and impactful experience, especially in times of loss, challenges, or crisis. The process of individual therapy is unique to every patient and similarly unique to the therapist. Most individual treatment sessions begin with a treatment contract. Once an individual is accepted into treatment, it is a good idea to make sure that your therapist is 100 percent committed to you and is working hard to relate to you in an authentic and genuine manner. Your recovery depends on how well your therapist can establish this connection with you, because it is a relationship that heals! I frequently remind myself of this in times when I find myself floundering, or focusing too much on improving my technique versus spending time building a trusting, therapeutic relationship with my patients. The process of individual therapy is just that, a process. Regardless of the therapeutic techniques used or even the mode of therapy itself, a psychotherapist's most valuable tool is the process that happens in a session with two individuals relating to one another. The conversation that begins with a patient during the first session is focused not on the content of the presenting problems (although it does play a role in case conceptualizations for therapists), but the process of *how* that content is being expressed. Psychotherapists then use this relational process to highlight everything of importance to a patient in the context of therapeutic work.

The process of individual therapy inevitably breeds process resistance in patients. It is difficult enough to be in therapy in the first place, but to be called out on the deepest and most difficult aspects of inner self can make individual weekly therapy appointments twice as challenging. Whereas group therapy is a place where confrontation of personal defenses and resistances appears once or twice a month based on the number of patients in a group, individual therapy allows for patients to examine their defenses almost on a weekly basis. Because of this, it is common for patients to experience intense emotions during sessions, since the defenses almost always tend to provoke anxiety. Patient's core issues are embedded within their resistances. I had a number of clients with issues of severe anxiety. One young boy, eleven years old, sat down and spent the session looking at the floor and refusing to say anything, almost daring me to make him answer my questions. A young woman in her thirties decided she would talk about everything under the sun, except her issues with anxiety, continuously pushing her chair away from me during the session. A middle-aged man would only discuss his anxiety issues when under pressure from his family, but otherwise would spend his one-hour session time looking at me to bring up material for therapy work. Although all three individuals came into therapy to address their issues with anxiety, none were able to initially discuss them, exhibiting behavioral defenses. Resistance is a necessary evil in individual therapy and is a central component of the therapeutic process. Although patients are often aware that they are engaging in unhelpful behaviors, few really understand how to break through the familiar patterns of functioning. The key role of a therapist is to identify and communicate those repetitive patterns to the patient and psychoeducate about how these patters shape a patient's present and future responses.

The process of resistance additionally puts patients in a position to hear therapist interpretations of their behaviors during the one-hour individual session time. During the hour, it would not be uncommon for a therapist to provide strength, supportive listening, and encouragement, while at the same time pointing out patient-related defenses. Treatment related discussions tend to force out material that challenges a particular patient's beliefs, thoughts, behaviors, and other resistances. Because these sessions can often lead patients to fall into further depression and anxiety or even invoke strong responses, an excellent therapist is adept at introducing the topic of resistance in such a way that patients would be willing to (1) hear it and (2) implement it. If timed correctly and done in a thoughtful manner, therapy can really take off with a patient, challenging his psychic equilibrium and encouraging a release of corresponding emotions. A helpful therapist will never push you on your resistances if you are neither ready nor able to process them. Remember, the point of therapy is to gain strength by becoming aware of your defenses and learning how to integrate those defenses. This process is extremely complex and requires some time and patience not only on the part of the patient, but also the treating clinician.

Perhaps the key to becoming comfortable with the process of individual therapy is the realization that it is essential for all of us to find ways to bring self-awareness into our everyday life. Psychotherapy is of course only one of many ways to expand self-awareness and is readily available to those who need it. Practicing yoga, taking a walk, biking, hiking, and spending time traveling would all be viable ways to enhance and explore our own working minds and experiences. Psychotherapy can be viewed as simply another vehicle of personal growth. I encourage many of my readers to find the answers they are looking for not only in an office with a professional, but also on the outside.

Just as I observe therapeutic success, I have also experienced an equal share of therapeutic failures or patients dropping out of therapy for one reason or another believing that it ultimately was not an avenue of change for them. One distinct memory is of a patient who came to see me for treatment of narcissistic personality disorder, although initially present with symptoms of depression. The patient was committed to building a successful career, and unfortunately through several years of building her business success had ultimately alienated her husband

and daughter. After a year of treatment, my patient mentioned to me that her daughter was home from college for the holidays and she wanted to bring her and her husband to the next session. When next week came, my patient was faced with two stern family faces, nervously waiting for what would happen next. My patient felt very reluctant to speak at first, but with a little encouragement from me, she began sharing with her husband and daughter her feelings of regret and guilt over her treatment of them over the years. She described specific instances for when she felt shame on the account of her behaviors and expressed regret and remorse for the time that was lost, and spent on fights and arguments. The patient's husband and daughter carefully listened and I slowly realized that they were not touched by what my patient had to say. They were soon arguing again and had left the office at odds with one another.

There are plenty of rich and satisfying rewards to being in therapy for every experience that does not necessarily end up in success. Therapeutic success may not happen every day, but it does occur, and when therapeutic goals are accomplished and success is reached, it is enough to keep you validated in your pursuits.

8

MEASURING THERAPEUTIC OUTCOMES

There are two possible outcomes: if the result confirms the hypothesis, then you have made a measurement. If the result is contrary to the hypothesis, then you have made a discovery.

—Enrico Fermi

Before walking through the door, every patient wants to know if the therapeutic process will be worth the time and the associated costs. This is an important question that deserves attention in this chapter. As I mentioned in a previous chapter, the ultimate vehicle of treatment success depends on a patient's own motivation level. However, there is another way to answer this question more in depth and is discussed next.

Psychotherapy, with all of its various theoretical orientations and approaches has been found to be effective across a variety of patient demographics ranging from different ages and disorders. This effectiveness has been researched over decades, including thousands of patients, settings, and cultural factors. The majority of research available supports the notion that psychotherapeutic treatments have been found to resolve pertinent distressing symptoms, interpersonal communication difficulties, and improve overall quality of life.[1] A specific percentage of success depends on the degree of symptom severity and motivation for treatment. In general, research shows that about two-thirds of patients get better with treatment, with only one-third showing regression in symptoms or exhibiting no benefit from treatment at all. With all available research, psychotherapy can be regarded as a positive, worthwhile experience for many, often resulting in reduction of presenting symptomatology. With that said, more improvement has yet to happen in many clinical settings, especially as it touches upon routine care.

Given the number of therapies and therapists out there, there has been little agreement on what specific therapeutic techniques are effective. An additional complication is, for example, that two therapists can use the same therapeutic technique with a different result. Such differences would dictate that many available therapeutic methods of practice are also a factor of training and experience. Unfortunately, many training programs that exist today vary in the diversity of their programs, and much disagreement about the type and extent of training that should be provided in psychological degree programs continues.

Recognizing that programs and training settings differ greatly in the type of programs that they offer, practitioners have agreed to provide treatment that is supported by scientific evidence. This treatment, also known as evidence-based practice (EBP), relies heavily on outcomes research. In recent years, a huge cultural shift occurred in the way consumers as well as clinicians view psychological treatment. Many patients that come for therapy do not regard therapy as a service with a fee, rather a commodity that can be bought based on positive treatment outcomes. As a result, many clinical settings have adopted use of measured outcomes, inviting patients to pay for what seems to work best in therapy. Historically, therapists have devoted a great deal of time and effort to refining and improving existent treatments versus assessing outcomes of the treatments they were already providing for patients. Attempts at measuring change is a fairly novel idea in the psychotherapeutic community, but it has generated a lot of data, systematically improving patient satisfaction and streamlining the entire psychotherapeutic process.

You may be wondering what outcomes data are and what do they measure specifically. In the psychotherapeutic process, outcomes data assess and measure areas such as depression, anxiety, or interpersonal difficulties. The existent measuring tools help assess symptoms relevant to a specific disorder. When a therapist selects a measuring tool, a particular domain is usually emphasized. The domains might include measuring and assessing a patient's cognitions, emotions, or behavior. However, a therapist will always use measuring devices that consider all three areas of change (i.e., cognition, emotion, and behavior). Measuring and monitoring changes in specific life domains allows therapists to adjust treatment as necessary when outcomes results point to lack of progress or treatment stasis.

Measuring patient progress is essential to providing routine care. In EBP studies, the assessments that were collected on patients for the purposes of improving care typically helped clinicians gather valuable patient feedback to target problematic domains. Given the serious issue of patient deterioration, dropout, and nonresponse to treatment, outcomes measures have become the standard in clinical care. For example, one such clinical tool and a central weekly measure of patient functioning is the Outcome Questionnaire-45 (OQ-45). The measuring tool was developed in 1993 and by 2001 became one of the self-report instruments for adults in routine care. This particular tool consists of forty-five questions, measuring patient functioning in broad areas. The OQ-45 is designed to be completed by patients each week prior to appointment time. Broadly speaking, completing the form takes anywhere between five and seven minutes, and the form is used to gather information on how well treatment is progressing. OQ-45 asks questions pertaining to symptoms of the presenting disorder, interpersonal functioning, as well as social functioning. All questions are scored on a scale of 0 to 4 yielding a total score ranging anywhere from 0 to 180. Scores in the higher range generally reveal problems in functioning in all three areas (i.e., exacerbation of symptoms, interpersonal and social problems).

As a derivative of OQ-45, another outcomes measure is S-OQ, which evaluates patient symptoms, capturing areas of severe psychopathology such as schizophrenia, bipolar disorder, and other psychotic illnesses. An S-OQ is a scale that is available to clinicians that includes questions assessing for severe disturbances and is a reasonable estimate of change for patients with the most severe diagnoses.

In addition to brief, weekly measures assessing and tracking treatment response in adults, other methods are available to monitor changes in adolescents and children. For example, the Y-OQ is a sixty-four-item questionnaire that measures symptoms and functioning in children ages four to seventeen. The Y-OQ is available in a form where parents and guardians can fill out the assessment as well, providing reliable data for children and adolescents. When comparing weekly answers of the Y-OQ between parents and children, the most common-ly observed difference is that children tend to underreport their behav-ioral issues, but are more accurate in regards to their internal states such as anxiety, depression, hopelessness, and loneliness, whereas parents and guardians are more accurate on the report of behavioral problems in school and at home. Each question on the Y-OQ specifically targets one of the major domain areas around interpersonal distress, social problems, behavioral issues, somatic complaints, and critical issues such as suicidal or homicidal thoughts, delusions, and eating disorder issues.

The basic assumption behind use of measured outcomes scales is to allow patients to provide feedback to clinicians. If a therapist understands and knows what works and what does not work, the targeted interventions, as well as the method of treatment can be improved. If we think about it, this is true for people in many areas of life, from learning how to play a sport or a musical instrument to education in general. Learning from feedback is intertwined with performance. If clinicians do not consider feedback worthwhile or even useful in the therapeutic process, the treatment will likely result in failure. Assessment tools can aid clinicians in understanding patient progress beyond what they might be able to do based on simply understanding a patient's situation or through observation alone. It is important that these assessment tools are added to treatment to enhance a psychotherapist's view of a patient's journey through change. An effective feedback system has to be immediate (before or after each session), frequent (weekly), and unambiguous (possibly containing graphic representations of patient progress). If such a system is utilized, both patient and clinician can view the treatment process as actual, versus what is hoped to be achieved.

Much like the monitoring systems already reviewed in this chapter, the others are constantly evolving such as the Clinical Outcomes in Routine Evaluation (CORE) system, AKQUASI system that has the advantage of offering additional measures in various languages, and COMPASS which reviews with patients their current well-being, symptoms, and life-functioning. Scores are calculated and summed in the Mental Health Index. The COMPASS system in particular is filled out by therapists and patients on a monthly basis throughout the course of treatment. Thus, using a variety of system monitoring techniques provides clinicians with valuable input on patient-related progress in therapy. Disadvantages of not using an outcomes-based method is the probability that 33 percent of patients will have terminated therapy after four weeks if clinicians are unable to discern poor outcomes in the initial stages of treatment.[2] Identifying red flags or cases at risk is crucial to enhancing positive outcomes.

The most significant problem to date with outcomes management systems is the high clinician resistance to using them. Psychotherapists think that they are effective most of the time as compared to their peers in the field. Many also believe that regardless of the outcomes, they would have helped most if not all of their patients. As a result, clinicians are resistant to using self-monitoring tools in therapy since it can be viewed as a weekly evaluation of effectiveness. Therefore when choosing a therapist, make sure that your patient needs are met by having your therapist use a treatment monitoring system that is a quick and easy evaluation of treatment progress and affirmation of money well spent.

Let me state the obvious and remind all my readers that just like any other service, psychotherapy is a business and should be viewed as such. Every business has a price tag and a typical client will be likely paying out of pocket for therapeutic services. It is obvious that faith alone should not keep any patient in psychotherapy, particularly if service costs are exceptionally high. According to a recent report, the number of mental health clinicians continues to be on the rise and it is clear that providers have to be increasingly competitive in the services that they deliver. The recent shift in paradigm where development of services was based purely on faith is no longer something that is in demand. In contemporary medical practices, there is little doubt that certain treatments will work based on supporting scientific research. As such, it is not surprising that this concept can and should be applied to therapy as well. After all, monitoring whether specific symptoms are subsiding based on a technique or a given theory of psychotherapy used is clearly something that can confirm the efficacy of any treatment. Thus EBP is not just a phrase that is frequently used to describe treatments that work, but is quickly becoming a mandated piece of clinical practice.

Other factors influencing treatment success that are common across all patient demographics and influence the course of therapy are family functioning and motivation. Interpersonal family functioning is an influential factor in treatment. Caregiver strain can also have an effect on patient participation in treatment. The associated increased stress, anxiety, and demand on raising a child with mental illness or behavioral issues have been tied to higher demand for mental health care.[3] Thus, parental involvement in the therapeutic process has been shown to have effects on clinical outcomes.

Much like family functioning, motivation and participation in therapy is another identified predictor of therapeutic success. Motivation and willingness to participate in treatment cannot be examined in the context of patient-related commitment to treatment, but can only be understood in the context of a therapeutic bond between a client and a therapist. I can generalize in stating that patient participation increases if a good match of services provided and a strong therapeutic connection with a particular clinician exists. Therapeutic alliance has been cited as one of the most effective components to successful outcomes in treatment.[4] A strong therapeutic alliance might play an even bigger role in adolescent and child mental health care. There are several reasons for why that is the case. First, a good therapeutic relationship between a therapist and a client, who is a minor, facilitates the necessary change mechanism that is the goal of therapy. Second, it functions as a thermometer in the interventions applied during treatment. Lastly, a good therapeutic relationship with a minor can affect outcomes in parental engagement. Treatment can focus on directly changing parental behaviors that affect a child's treatment, provide adherence to treatment and appointment attendance, and promote relevant treatment gains outside therapy sessions. It is thus important to consider that a good therapeutic bond between a therapist and a child is predictive of symptom improvement, and subsequently opens the possibility for greater patient participation in treatment.

Controlled, measured treatment in therapy should be a standard among all mental health clinicians. Regular therapist feedback can allow for identification of patients who are "at-risk" for treatment failure, and implementation of changes for attainment of positive outcomes. Monitored feedback can also result in keeping those patients in therapy who can benefit from longer treatment, and shorten the stay of those who are on track for successful outcomes. Remember that outcomes-informed clinical care will not help patients unless gathered often as the treatment process progresses. Additionally, knowing what works gives patients the knowledge necessary in determining which curative factors work, and which fall short of producing the necessary benefits. In short, an uninformed treatment is a waste of time and money, where neither the therapist nor the patient understand exactly what works and what does not. When choosing a therapist, please remember that your frequent input is crucial to the integrated success of care. Moreover, your participation in the therapy process matters greatly in the type of care that you will ultimately be receiving. I invite you to be an advocate for the best possible care, which you deserve, and modify treatment as needed to get what you want.

9

ADVANTAGES AND DISADVANTAGES OF INSURANCE

The first wealth is health.

—Ralph Waldo Emerson

If you ever had an opportunity to attend a professional psychology or psychiatry conference, you will find that many members are angry when it comes to managed care. You may have read online that managed care compromises patients' welfare. While the current system of managed care may fall short of expectations, the issue to discuss is whether healthcare management represents a step in the right direction. This chapter explores the numerous existent payment options available in outpatient treatment and also discusses advantages and disadvantages of insurance use for mental health treatment.

In addition to adopting the new demands of measurable outcomes in therapy, therapists must also consider working with managed care companies for more patients to consider outpatient therapy and to be able to afford associated costs. Currently, there exist many ways to afford individual outpatient treatment even if fees are high. Generally, available options include sliding scale, insurance use, fluctuating fee options, and a no-fee possibility. For starters, let's explore the sliding scale option. Every therapist with an outpatient practice has a sliding scale available to patients. A sliding scale is a common fee arrangement between a therapist and his patients. This particular option allows patients to afford therapy by paying what they can based on an individually tailored plan worked out in collaboration with a therapist. In addition to a private practice option, patients can receive more sliding scale information from specific clinics and agency settings that allow patients to explore payment methods based on income and other factors. One of the primary concerns with a sliding scale option is that some patients may present a certain financial picture just to obtain a lower fee. This can be a problem if the fee structure is not established early on in the therapeutic process and can cause strain on the therapeutic relationship. In practice, however, this occurs rarely since a therapist will set a fee agreement before the start of therapy.

Another option available that many are not aware of is a "no-fee service." Most ethics boards and authors have advocated for years for a no-fee arrangement with those patients that truly cannot afford the fees of services. Many clinicians in private practice can allow themselves a small percentage of patients under a "no-fee agreement," especially if a clinician is conducting university or hospital-affiliated research that has the potential to benefit both interested parties. Organizations such as the Veterans' Administration, counties, and correctional facility sites provide free therapy to patients, given that the patient can demonstrate that he is unable to afford service fees.

The most popular way to afford therapy, however, is through health insurance. Most health insurance and managed care companies require a copayment from the patient, which is an additional amount to the payment that will be covered by insurance. Many restrictions go along with using insurance to cover the costs of therapy. Those restrictions include but are not limited to length of treatment and ability to choose a therapist of your own choice. These restrictions will be discussed later on in this chapter.

A final option of coverage that patients can consider fits under the heading of "fluctuating fees." Suppose you have started the therapy process and in the course of six months have lost your job, health insurance, and are suddenly facing serious financial troubles. In this case, hopefully your therapist is open and understanding to the situation and is flexible with payment accommodations. Now, of course, therapists themselves have to make a living and are not all agreeable to fluctuating fees. With that in mind, there are circumstances where treatment warrants further consideration and is in the interest and ethical obligation of every therapist, even under patient financial duress.

Having discussed all relevant payment options, there still exists a prevalent view that patients who pay more, benefit from therapy more, based on the high costs associated with treatment. Cultural norms would dictate that "free cheese is only in the mouse trap" and "you get what you pay for" mentality. Some people go even further in their thinking and assume that the higher the cost of services, the more qualified the clinician providing those services. These and other cultural notions have not been supported by research and very little indication exists to suggest that those who engage in no-cost therapy benefit any less from services rendered. In fact, the only available research suggests that the outcome and success of therapy depends on the therapeutic relationship between a patient and his therapist and the level of motivation that a patient has to reach therapeutic goals.[1]

What are the benefits of paying for your psychotherapy versus using insurance? The number one reason that people choose to pay out of pocket for therapy is privacy. Whenever insurance is used to cover the cost of psychotherapy, not all information can be kept private. Generally, insurance companies will ask for detailed patient information before covering costs of treatment. This information consists of personal patient demographics, along with a diagnosis, which at times is made available to employers. When you pay out of pocket, your privacy is completely protected from managed care companies and insurance companies. Third parties are entirely eliminated from the equation, leaving you with the sole decision of who you may want to share your medical information with at no loss of privacy. An additional benefit to paying out of pocket is the ability to keep your diagnosis private, or not have a "diagnosis" in the paperwork altogether. Whenever insurance is used in the process of psychotherapy, treatment has to be deemed as medically necessary, which means that your treating clinician *must* give you a diagnosis. When patients pay out of pocket, they can request that a formal diagnosis be kept out of treatment, thereby ensuring that a "label" of a particular mental illness does not follow them for the rest of their lives. Some patients view leaving out a diagnosis from treatment as a necessary and effective factor in the psychotherapeutic process, thus relieving themselves from judgmental third-party reviews undermining their sense of privacy. Many use therapy to help themselves deal with difficult life transitions, marital problems or simply personal growth, and not necessarily chronic, severe psychological issues. Taking the diagnosis out of treatment ensures that a patient does not have to deal with the effects of a label to receive mental health care.

At the heart of any diagnosis is a conceptualization of what constitutes a disorder based on criteria as defined in the *Diagnostic and Statistical Manual of Mental Disorders* (DSM-5). The specific criteria of disorders define individual dysfunction based on level of distress and disability. It might be interesting for readers to realize that the psychiatric diagnostic system as it stands today is a simple product of historical accident. The DSM was originally a compilation of observed mental and behavioral phenomena that could be grouped together based on reasonable assumptions. As a result, the current distributed diagnoses are a product that exists because a group of professionals decided to categorize mental illness in defined and concrete terms versus actually conducting rational, research driven study design.[2] What frequently happens in therapy then is that two different people with supposed two different diagnostic labels have to learn the same skills in therapy. Although advertised under a different heading (i.e., depression versus paranoia), a depressed client has to learn how to reframe his negative thinking style, just as a paranoid client who is ruminating on different possible future outcomes has to learn ways to cope with negative thinking. Therefore, it can be misleading to think that different diagnostic labels lead to different therapy needs, as well as different insurance coverage needs. While a diagnosis can always give a treating clinician valuable information on certain upcoming treatment challenges, it can be easy to miss the fact that patients with different diagnostic labels can and do often confront similar problems.

Most people seeking outpatient psychotherapy do not have an actual diagnosis. Recent research has indicated that in general, people entering outpatient care have only a mild psychiatric disorder, with 60 percent not qualifying for a formal psychiatric diagnosis.[3] In recent years, a growing debate continues over when psychotherapy is medically necessary and when it is only an activity that has the potential to improve efficacy in certain life areas. Attempts by clinicians to justify reimbursement through insurance companies are what made it partially necessary to fit a patient into a defined diagnostic label. Ultimately it can be argued that even presenting cases of mild distress should be covered through insurance, given that alleviated stress can reduce overall cost of

health care, saving insurance companies money over time. Unfortunately, many healthcare companies define mental health care in terms of
their bottom line. If a given outpatient treatment method can save
money by not sending a patient into a hospital, it makes sense to cover
costs and write it off as a sound short-term investment. Thus, the majority of those patients seeking outpatient care by using insurance fall prey
to labeling practices that do not always communicate accurately the
degree or severity of a particular presenting problem. These patients
are almost always pathologized, which can lead to stigma and a distorted
perception of treatment itself.

For more than thirty years, clinicians have struggled with increasing
the use of diagnoses for coverage purposes. Third parties can restrict
mental health coverage to those that are deemed "medically necessary."
Many insurance policies only cover diagnoses that are listed under the
Axis I category, which by definition include cases that are difficult to
treat and would remit after a certain time. Problems with diagnostic
labels are twofold. First, diagnostic overuse dilutes the amount of useful
information that can and should be used for patients who actually have
debilitating symptoms. Second, a diagnostic label reinstates a patient's
view of their problems as "abnormal." I would go even further to say
that a diagnostic label can hamper a patient's ability to implement
changes, transforming a treatment experience into a label of "sickness"
versus symptoms that can be helped with a definitive set of behaviors
and thinking patterns.

Although insurance use is a popular way of payment for therapy,
another disadvantage that patients have to consider is the ability to
choose your preferred therapist. Unfortunately, when insurance companies are involved in paying for treatment, they often limit the choices
of therapists. Many times, the available network of providers is quite
good and allows patients to receive quality treatment from clinicians
who make it their responsibility to provide the best services possible
without sacrificing the quality of treatment based on certain loyalties to
insurance companies. At other times, however, clinicians are unable to
put patient needs first based on existent obligations to third-party providers. A typical example of a conflict may be a client presenting for
treatment with a diagnosis of moderate depression. His particular insurance only covers ten treatment sessions. The therapist takes on this
client knowing in advance that depression may not be resolved in ten

sessions with this particular client; however, he provides a brief treatment model nonetheless. When a patient does not experience treatment benefits after ten sessions and is unable to pay for future therapy sessions, the therapist promptly concludes treatment. This is a common example of what sometimes can occur when patients use insurance to pay for psychotherapy, placing the patient as well as the therapist, at a deep disadvantage for providing and receiving quality care.

Insurance use in mental health care can also have an effect on the length of treatment. In previous chapters I discussed the various existent theories and models of care ranging from Freudian psychoanalytic treatment to brief treatment modalities such as CBT. Managed care companies often limit the type of treatment that patients can receive. As a standard, brief-solution focused therapeutic modalities are preferred over lengthy types of treatment that rely heavily on psychoanalysis. Working more incisively can be threatening to many patients and therapists, particularly those who adhere to more conservative psychoanalytic treatment methods. Many would caution against brief psychoanalysis, simply because many patients are fragile and briefer modalities challenge ways in which clinicians can take advantage of time and have the flexibility necessary to handle this fragility.

While some insurance companies can interfere very little with the choice and type of treatment, others make important decisions, which include the type of therapy available and the length of treatment for specific presenting concerns. Therefore some patients consider paying out of pocket to ensure that they receive the type and length of treatment that is most appropriate for their particular needs.

The next question relevant to most readers of this book is "Is psychotherapy a wise way to spend money?" If using insurance to cover costs of treatment does not necessarily provide you with the type of therapist or treatment that you may want or need, then is paying out of pocket a wise investment of your time and money? When people ultimately decide to see a psychotherapist, in my opinion, the improvements they make in their lives often result in financial success. How does therapy lead to financial benefits? Well, for starters, one clear financial benefit is reduced medical expenses. Research frequently shows that many people suffer health-related concerns due to untreated stress or other mental health issues. When left untreated, mental health issues can and do result in people taking time off from work, using sick days, or even not feeling as productive as they once were in their daily lives. Problems in relationships and family lives can be equally taxing, further increasing healthcare expenses through unplanned doctor and emergency room visits. Issues in relationships often result in depression, anxiety, and sometimes even panic attacks. Fortunately, employers are becoming increasingly aware of mental health concerns amongst workers, with employees exhibiting low productivity at high financial costs. People from all walks of life are beginning to see the benefits of psychotherapy with results often showing spikes in effectiveness and performance. Current research studies show that overall medical cost savings are significant. When costs were measured over a period of five years among thousands of subjects studied, therapy resulted in overall decrease in healthcare costs.[4]

When is treatment cost effective from the patient's point of view? When treatment allows patients to complete their education rather than flunk out; or avoid relationship stress such as a divorce; or to be more efficient and productive at work due to less stress or anxiety, psychotherapy becomes a gratifying process and a means to a satisfying end. According to the National Alliance on Mental Illness (NAMI), 70 percent of those diagnosed with a psychiatric illness rank work as an important priority for themselves. Mental health counseling helps more than 50 percent of patients find stable employment, providing support and intensive outpatient reach programs. Work becomes the center of life for most people, providing purpose, financial freedom, identity, and meaning. There is a need to recognize that psychotherapy can and does affect work productivity, family, and marital satisfaction, as well as people's overall satisfaction with life. Studies show that those that have gone into therapy have felt happier and more productive, with a significant decrease in depression, anger, fatigue, tension, and other somatic complaints.

When estimating the financial benefits of therapy, look at whether psychotherapy has the potential to lower your depression, anxiety, or stress over a certain period, and thereby affect possible changes in employment, promotions, family relationships, or academic education. Considering these factors and weighing the pros and cons of receiving mental health treatment may justify the investment in psychotherapy. Moreover, certain intangible improvements cannot be measured, but can equally affect your quality of life. These improvements may involve your overall satisfaction and happiness level. Just like with any other investment, psychotherapy has to be considered through a lens of benefits and losses. Evaluating whether your problems can be improved through therapy while bearing in mind costs can, in the long term, help you avoid expensive medical bills and other related concerns such as job performance and individual or family issues.

10

FAMILY THERAPY

The principle aim of psychotherapy is not to transport one to an impossible state of happiness, but to help acquire steadfastness and patience in the face of suffering.

—C. G. Jung

For those looking to begin family therapy, I devote a chapter discussing the ins and outs of an integrative family therapy approach as a theoretical model of family therapy. Interestingly, many individuals start therapy by coming in for individual weekly sessions, which can at times evolve into family therapy. Patients ask what family therapy is all about and how one therapist can possibly address the needs of the entire family in a one-hour weekly session. This of course begs the question: "What is family therapy?"

Family therapy begins by searching for the meaning of human behavior. A therapist may ask herself: "Why is this family experiencing dysfunction, depression, or anxiety?" As previously discussed, all therapists adopt therapy models to explain the human condition in the therapeutic context. Whether these explanations are rooted in behavioral, cognitive, or social systems is somewhat irrelevant, since they all attempt to understand the same thing—human behavior.

Family therapy, much like other brief therapy modality models is well structured with an average length of ten to fifteen sessions per family. The therapist organizes the session according to tasks and stages, moving through them in a systematic manner toward termination. Clearly, no therapeutic process can always move in an organized fashion; therefore, any theoretical model that a therapist uses has to provide for some flexibility during the live session. For a therapist, a theoretical orientation is essential to structure and organize the sometimes disorganized and chaotic presentation of ideas and feelings in families. A family in conflict can especially benefit from structure, as not every member can always rationally evaluate what each is saying or doing. A therapist, who has a strong theoretical process, will always establish order within chaos, and guide the session in such a way that each member's goals are met.

A typical structure of therapy with families has five organized stages. The first important organization stage is structure. A therapist asserts control from the beginning regarding a particular problematic situation. A therapist in this capacity has to introduce herself to the family with warmth, acceptance, and care, while concurrently tackling the human drama of each family's life. A therapist must always maintain objectivity and separateness to allow for a productive therapeutic encounter in each session. To establish structure, a therapist begins by setting a definitive length, time, and frequency of sessions. It is important for the structure of family therapy that each member attend the first several sessions for a therapist to observe the interaction, as well as gather the necessary assessment information.

The second task for any therapist working with families is to make a connection with each individual member. This particular task is tricky, insofar as the therapist should be able to communicate concerns for the entire family as well as each individual within the family. Moreover, a therapist should lead each family member to feel the importance of his contribution to the family unit for the overall success of the family relationship.

A third task is for the therapist to model a healthy communication process. A seasoned therapist has to be very clear and specific when interacting with families and encourage each member to behave in this way also. Often in the throes of a heated debate, family members forget to listen and communicate appropriately with one another. The task of a therapist is to make sure that each member's needs, feelings, and statements are communicated in a clear and concise manner, teaching family members to give feedback to one another, and asking for clarification when others' statements are misunderstood or misinterpreted. The outlined three tasks are critical to a successful beginning of any family therapy. In a sense, a therapist builds a productive therapeutic relationship with each member of the family in the beginning, while concurrently asserting control, building structure, and setting the stage for later therapeutic changes.

Family therapy continues with the next stage that involves observation and assessment. A therapist takes two sessions to evaluate the general dynamics within the family, as well as each individual. The first step is an evaluation of specific problems that have brought the family into therapy. These problems can and should be translated into short-term goals for the family. As assessment moves on further, some longer-term goals can be outlined to better address the presenting concerns. The completed assessment, as well as short-term and long-term goals, are shared with the family upon completion of the initial evaluation period. The therapist can additionally present therapeutic goals in order of importance, letting the family decide whether they agree with the evaluation. Once the assessment is out of the way, a therapist determines present and future interventions and shares with the family an outline for therapy, allowing each member to accept or modify the proposed treatment plan.

Based on the diagnostic picture that is developed in the second stage of treatment, a therapist begins to identify specific techniques that will ultimately institute change within the family. The intervention list that a therapist can choose from is exhaustive; however, the major intervention strategies address the presenting concerns, identify confrontation techniques to help members communicate more effectively with one another, and work out definite roles and expectations for each member in the family. Additional techniques involve communication checks to ensure that family members understand and perceive each other correctly, as well as a set of guidelines that can help facilitate healthy interactions for all family members. Almost all therapists, regardless of therapeutic orientation, use these major techniques. They are not the only therapeutic tools, and thus all therapists have their own repertoire to supplement the process of change.

The primary focus of the next stage in family therapy is reinforcement of new patterns of interaction learned during the previous stage. At this stage, a therapist will generally increase the time between sessions, to remove himself from a central position within the family, and allow each member to incorporate new insights, behaviors, and cognitions into conflict resolution. The family at this point is actively involved in solving its own issues with continued, infrequent input from the therapist.

The final stage in the family therapy process is termination and review of skills learned for better problem solving. A therapist ensures that each member's goals for therapy have been addressed and the family has internalized new behaviors and attitudes around problem solving. The final task of the therapist is to present written and verbal feedback to the family regarding the therapeutic process, including a discussion of the initial presenting problem, assessment, members' goals, and review of present functioning. Readers of this book should always make sure that their therapist presents and follows a set structure when conducting therapy. This structure should be applicable not only to family therapy, but also to individual and group therapy formats. Successful therapy always follows a progression from structuring to termination, with all the fun intervening stages in the middle of the process.

The following example shows how a therapist may work with a family from the initial assessment session to termination. Let's take a family and consider how it can benefit from a few sessions with a family therapist. Our family will be the Joneses consisting of Mike Jones, fifty-nine, his wife Carol Jones, fifty-three, Bill, seventeen, who is Mike's son from a previous marriage, and Judy, fifteen, who is Mike and Carol's daughter. The Joneses are a middle-class family who live in the suburbs of a large city. Mike is an insurance agent and Carol is a surgical nurse. Bill attends a local high school, where he plays football, and Judy is in the band, attending the same school. Since the time Bill was very young, he lived with his mother and spent weekends with his father. Approximately five years ago, legal custody was changed because Bill's mother was having financial issues and Bill came to live with his father full time.

Mike contacted a family therapist, requesting counseling for his son Bill, who has been having problems at school, nearly failing all of his classes, and skipping football practices on a regular basis. Mike felt that therapy would allow Bill to express some of his anger in regards to the current living arrangement, as well as allow the family to work out their individual differences and improve communication. Mike mentioned that he and his wife Carol were currently having issues and were seeing a couple's counselor on a weekly basis.

The initial session with a family therapist begins with an introduction to the process of therapy. Bill was asked to expand on his relationship with his half-sister, biological mother, and stepmother. After a few minutes of gathering information, it was clear that Bill felt detached from the rest of the family, pointing out that he did not feel very connected to Judy or Carol, mentioning that a relationship with them was almost nonexistent. Bill's circle of support consisted of a few friends from school that were twenty minutes away from his house by car. Bill admitted to feeling unmotivated to attend football practice after school and nearly failing almost all of his classes. Although ordinarily viewed as a B-average student, Bill was currently getting almost all Ds. Bill felt that he was not getting enough support or encouragement at home and felt that everything that came out of his dad's mouth was a criticism. Listening to Bill describe their relationship, Mike admitted to feeling stressed, sharing that he and Carol have been working with a couple's counselor to address the issue of how to better communicate with Bill.

During the second session, Mike discussed his relationship with Carol and termed the relationship as just "ok." Mike discussed that they were not together much of the time because of work schedules, kids, and other obligations. Mike additionally discussed that he felt Carol left most of the parenting responsibilities of Bill to him. He thought that Carol did not want to attempt to drive a wedge between them by taking sides, and thus stayed out of things for the most part. Mike shared that he wished Carol had been more involved with Bill, and at times was very angry with her for not taking care of her end of parenting responsibilities. Bill was additionally questioning expectations that he had for himself. Bill reported that he wanted to be successful, to graduate high school, and go to a good college. When asked why he would set those expectations for himself, Bill reported that he mainly wanted to get out of his dad's house and start living his own life. The first homework assignment was to have each family member work on their individual short-term and long-term goals for therapy.

After completion of the first two sessions, a therapist takes the time to write out an integrative evaluation, summarizing family themes, individual dynamics, role expectations, and communicational patterns within the family. In the case discussed, a therapist's evaluation might begin by focusing on the structural dynamics within the family such as: rigid boundaries between Mike and Carol in regards to parenting, conflict in the parental unit, and Bill's isolation from the family. In terms of role expectations for the family, a therapist might highlight to the Joneses a lack of clear expectations from the children and lack of consequences or follow-through action by all family members. Certain patterns of communication within the family have to be evaluated also, where the blame statements made by Mike and Bill as well as the defensive nature of the words created a blocked perception by all members. To underline particular family themes, a therapist might mention to the Joneses that they cannot appear to negotiate their differences within the blended family unit, perpetuating the continued interpersonal conflict.

After the initial integrative evaluation is completed, in the third session, a therapist will complete the family assessment, providing important information to the family on the commitment to work on mutually agreed-upon goals. A possible homework assignment might be for Mike and Carol to work on mutual parental expectations and Bill to set some short-term goals for himself in regards to his grades and attendance at football practices. Subsequent sessions focus on the therapist intervening with the family to address therapy goals.

Every family runs into its set of problems and no family is exempt. One of the most important family responsibilities is the task of learning and teaching. The family becomes a vehicle for communicating and teaching knowledge and skills that are then passed onto younger generations. The learning process begins early and parents start to pass down knowledge to sons and daughters in their infancy. As time goes on, the children eventually teach their parents about new ways of thinking and behaving. The openness with which this process can take place is exactly what defines family functioning and health. Attempting to set up a healthy development of a family involves a number of factors that include support, stability, privacy, independence, problem solving, and a defined set of expectations. A therapist's role is the promotion of these factors to help create mutuality and trust amongst all family members.

In sessions, the task of defining expectations appears to be most critical when working with families. When family members have unrealistic expectations for one another, it becomes a source of discontent and unhappiness. The emphasis of psychotherapy then is to help members create reasonable and realistic expectations for one another on a daily basis. Members are taught to ask themselves how likely certain goals will be accomplished, and what the time is within which those goals can and will be reached. This is more likely to occur in a setting where the family atmosphere is open for discussion and there is an air of mutual decision-making. This type of commitment from all family members is a difficult process and sometimes requires quite a bit of work in therapy.

The problem-solving process in every family is another key to health and well functioning. A therapist will look at how problems are defined and resolved in the present and whether the methods are effective. A therapist will examine whether a family has set up a system where the problem-solving process is rigid and does not tolerate any flexibility or is open to feedback from other members and is solution focused. More often than not, the way in which a family handles insignificant day-to-day problems is exactly what defines how that family handles major conflict. Teaching families how to handle small issues with flexibility and openness is one of the major aspects to family therapy.

A related issue to the provision of health and functioning in families is stability. Families often present to therapy not having defined any type of family structure for all family members. This type of environment can be confusing for children, and thus prevents them from getting used to a particular type of routine. When working with families, therapists will often inquire into a family structure that exists within the home, and whether children have a permanent living arrangement, set bedtimes, consistent mealtimes, and factors that help promote structure. An absence of this type of structure leads families to present to an initial session arguing with one another over issues of responsibility and division of labor. If a particular family lacks structure and consistency, a therapist will work with the family on establishing common goals that could let members know how they can depend on others for structure. An established routine can also encourage independence of each family member, which is crucial for a healthy self-concept and development.

Thus if the family chooses to seek professional help, the therapeutic interventions will target the areas of support, stability, independence, expectations, and problem solving. A clinician will first identify the dysfunction, and then help the family make changes through the therapeutic process. This process may be short or long depending on the way

family members relate to one another and solve problems. As the therapy draws to an end, members can learn strategies to deal with stress in
the future. The discussion of the nature of family health and growth is
largely theoretical; however, it can give readers a feel for what happens
to a family when members are experiencing difficulty and what can be
expected in terms of therapeutic interventions. Many times, families
come into therapy as a last ditch effort to resolve conflict. A therapist is
left to untangle what can be viewed as years of "dysfunction." Family
members should understand that the dysfunction cannot be changed
overnight and in some cases, years of effort have to be expended to
achieve results. Therefore, in any family work, keep in mind the goal of
looking forward to the day when family members can picture themselves as healthy and functioning in the family dynamic. Successful
family therapy almost always follows the progression from stages of
disappointment, pain, and drama to that of excitement and satisfaction.
Therefore, keep in mind the end goal when going through all the initial
stages.

11

PROJECTIONS AND RESISTANCE IN THERAPY

Men are more moral than they think and far more immoral than they can imagine.

—Sigmund Freud

With the first therapeutic encounter, as you walk through the door, a bond begins to develop. This bond in psychotherapy is precisely what is necessary for treatment success between a therapist and a patient. Recognizing this fact, healing begins to take place, firmly placing the process of feelings into the safety of the relationship. The feelings are often raw and unprocessed, leaving the patient vulnerable to the phenomenon of transference. I will not discuss the endless descriptions of transference found in any contemporary text of psychoanalytic literature. I will simply state that transference is a process by which a patient transfers feelings onto the therapist, especially where figures from a patient's life are likely to be idealized or despised. The difficulty and the task during the session for the therapist is to sort out what might be issues pertinent to the present day and those that are vested heavily in the past with a bearing on the present. When a patient displays overt hostility, love, frustration, anger, or any emotionally charged reaction, transference is considered carefully.

Transference feelings that occur in the therapeutic relationship are a result of a number of psychological exchanges that occur over the course of treatment. The nature of a patient's powerful feelings may be a result of an imagined connection or believed behavior or intent on the part of the therapist, which is not supported by the therapists' actual actions or words. This is of course a normal and expected response in therapy. In the early days of psychoanalysis, many psychoanalysts were surprised that their patients had begun "falling in love" with them. Some were even alarmed to have discovered the existence of such strong feelings. However, with time and good progress in therapy, the patient eventually learns to expose these intense feelings for what they are, and the therapeutic relationship continues to grow. Alarmingly, in recent years, the response of some therapists to their patients' romanticized feelings toward them has been inappropriate and various books and articles warn patients of sexual abuse in the therapeutic relationship. Notably, some patients' feelings are not that of love but of extreme hate, leaving the therapist just as responsible for an appropriate, professional response.

Not every psychotherapeutic exchange that occurs in the process of therapy is of a transferential nature. Arguably every level of exchange that occurs in the room is different based on the patient, emotional activity, and the level of experience that a therapist possesses. A competent therapist has to differentiate a patient's emotionally charged response from that of a transaction involving a patient's own material involving the sometimes projected feelings rooted in the past toward the therapist. To give a reader a chance to understand what transference may look like in the therapeutic process, I will describe an imagined situation involving a woman who comes in for treatment of anxiety, stress, and depression.

CASE STUDY I

Stephanie, a woman in her mid-thirties, with a career, marriage, and two young children comes into therapy complaining of high levels of stress, exhaustion, depression, and frequent anxiety. After eight months of therapy, Stephanie's marriage dissolves; however, she is able to focus on her career and flourishes as an independent, driven business woman. Stephanie's children are adjusting to the new life of sharing their time between two households and Stephanie is juggling life as a single mother. During holiday time, Stephanie comes into session with a bright smile on her face, holding a very expensive gift. She presents the gift to her therapist, explaining that she is grateful to have found someone so understanding, giving, and caring, and would be lost if it weren't for the weekly therapy sessions. As the session proceeds, Stephanie is flashing attractive smiles toward the therapist. The therapist accepts the gift and wishes Stephanie a happy holiday season, until the following session. The gift is appropriate, albeit a bit expensive (a large, decorative box of chocolates). The boundary confusion is exposed when the therapist realizes that he does not have a gift for his patient, and accepted his usual weekly fee along with the gift after the session ends. The therapist takes time to process the session and sets up target goals for the following week, deciding to initiate a discussion on the nature of the relationship with the patient and the meaning behind the gift.

This is a typical way in which transference could manifest itself during treatment. The patient may have experienced feelings of gratitude toward the therapist, and thus wanted to honor those feelings with a holiday gift. Nevertheless, the possibility cannot be excluded that the present may also have been suggestive of the depth of attachment she felt toward the therapist. Given the nature of her presenting concerns, Stephanie lost a rather important relationship in her life, her husband, and may have been discovering feelings toward her therapist to replicate her possible unfulfilled emotional needs. Given the possibility of transference, the responsibility of the therapist is then to explore further with the patient if the emotional transference was indeed present. The therapist can then proceed to draw attention to the patients' lost relationships and set limits on her relationship with the therapist. If the therapist does not take the time to consider the possibility of transference, the patient may take a long while before embracing another heterosexual relationship, which can continue to fuel her anger toward her ex-husband who deserted the family. Until the therapist-patient relationship is again realistic versus idealistic, the patient risks the chance of disillusionment both in therapy and outside.

The difficulty for the therapist is that transference manifests itself in many ways. Sometimes it is easy to pick out and identify and at other times patients' feelings are only obvious during a particularly intense session, where emotions well up to the forefront for both the patient and the therapist. The feelings can even manifest themselves in strong dislike, betrayal, or anger, all intense and powerful negative emotions. The issue of transference is thus a continuing theme in the psychotherapeutic process, which can at times lead many therapists to experience strong emotions toward their patients which are not otherwise substantiated by any real behavioral or verbal encounters. The approach to handling transference clinically can be challenging and often requires consultation. If unmanaged, the consequences can be dire and potentially disconcerting clinically. A colleague's objective perspective can at times be necessary to steer a truer course for a therapist that is struggling with intense, transferential experiences.

I mentioned earlier that therapists can also experience strong emotive reactions toward their patients. We call this phenomenon countertransference, which is very similar to the experience of the patient, only in reverse. The therapist is left managing their own reactions to a particular patient, that may not be based in the reality of the relationship, but rooted in past interactions or traumas for the therapist. The following is an example of an imagined encounter between a therapist and her patient, with the therapist struggling to reconcile her own emotions in session.

CASE STUDY 2

A female therapist finds herself to be angry and a bit dismissive of her male patient. The patient is a strong, opinionated businessman, willing to express his feelings on subjects in a forceful way. The female therapist respects her patient's way of being able to express himself as well as his forward nature, but finds it difficult to work with him on the weekly basis. The therapist perceives her patient to be an ungrateful man, who is going through a difficult time both financially and personally, but is also giving her a hard time for no justifiable reason. The male patient additionally tested boundaries earlier in treatment and has a bad habit of being consistently late for appointments. The latter was particularly upsetting for the therapist and she discovered herself to be angry with the patient before their sessions. When the anger became consistent, the therapist dug deep into her own personal experiences and the feelings she had toward strong, authoritative men. After some time, the therapist realized that her anger raised issues that touched on helplessness, control, and power with strong male figures. Her own father would assert control each day by giving orders and demanding excellence in academics and everywhere else. The therapist's own fears appeared as she grew up in an atmosphere of tension and oppression. Later in life, the therapist learned to convert those same feelings of fear into anger. Some of the anger was felt toward her father, as she never understood why he was so tough on her growing up, and some was her own anxiety at having to deal with demanding and controlling male figures.

The critical patient, completely unaware of the feelings the therapist was experiencing, was entering into dangerous territory. If left unmanaged, countertransference can mean the end of therapy. Unless the therapist takes time for self-reflection and awareness, along with needed supervision, the therapy will be directed against the patient. "Counter" in this sense, simply means that the therapist is moving away from the patient and away from the relationship necessary for treatment to succeed. The example described here demonstrates precisely how powerful a therapist's unresolved issue can be for the patient. Thus, careful monitoring of the infinite variety of transference and countertransference phenomena that appear in the course of treatment is by far the most exciting and challenging part of the therapeutic endeavor.

There is a feeling that we all experience upon meeting a stranger for the first time. Whether a casual encounter or a meeting of a professional nature, we all have a response to new people in our lives. This feeling is not anything that can be defined in words or rationally explained. Most people would recognize this gut response, where the unconscious is activated and you are ready to take the plunge, regardless of what your brain tells you to do in the moment. Walking through the door for your first session is much like that feeling. You have thoughts, feelings, and judgments about the process and yet, you are also willing to trust your gut response about the stranger that sits before you. This feeling is strong and can be either positive or negative; however, the significance of that response is what will ultimately sway you to stay or go.

CASE STUDY 3

A new patient, Suzie, stood in the doorway extending her hand. Her face did not give in by way of much information. She appeared tense and looked a bit angry. Much to my own surprise, Suzie's angry look did not stir any feelings in me and the moment before I invited her to step into the office, I felt a wave of relief and hope in being able to work with this woman. Because Suzie looked tense, I tried hard to suppress a big welcome smile and instead sat down getting the usual business of the first session out of the way. Suzie made herself comfortable on the couch, crossing her legs, with a look of suspicion in her eyes. We took a moment to look at each other and not say much. Looking at Suzie, I explained that the first few sessions will be for assessment purposes only and invited her to tell me why she came into therapy. There was another prolonged silence before Suzie felt comfortable enough to speak. Then, quite unexpectedly she began her account of how much she despised the field of clinical psychology and was sick and tired of all the therapists that she had seen in the past. She ended her long speech by adamantly stating: "I no longer believe in this process and hate sitting here across from you not knowing once again if this will work for me." A response came to me almost immediately as I listened to her: "Well that much is obvious from the minute you shook my hand." We gave each other a long look and burst out laughing.

As soon as Suzie walked through the door, I had a feeling about her that was relaxed and comfortable. I felt in a single instance that I could like this woman and work with her effectively. Suzie did not mince words, and after the first session, we both came to a tentative conclusion that her journey in treatment would not be an easy one, but that she was willing to try. It is hard to explain why you have reactions toward certain people that make it somewhat easier to work with them. Suzie did not want to come into therapy and was reluctant to start the therapeutic work. Any other therapist may have met Suzie's reaction with hesitation and labeled her as yet "another difficult patient." I behaved spontaneously and trusted my inner response to Suzie and continued working productively with her week in and week out, trusting that Suzie will make progress. Many times, patients walk into a therapist's office reluctant to try therapy, and sometimes it is only that gut feeling about the process or the therapist that can help make the determination in a patient's mind to either give therapy a try or give up altogether. Suzie and I worked productively for a few months and eventually parted ways with a mutual feeling of satisfaction.

As you begin psychotherapeutic work, the "rules" you have to follow are not always easy. You may not agree with these rules, and some are just plain difficult to follow based on your notion of what is "right" for you in the moment. One such rule is the subject of self-disclosure. When you begin uncovering your psychic processes and doing the therapeutic work, disclosure is not always possible; however, therapists will ask that you avoid all personal censorship, keeping in mind the limits of confidentiality. Disclosure has to be agreed on by the patient to build toward openness and trust in the relationship with a therapist. Having said that, disclosure does not always occur in therapy and the "right" therapist has to discern and carefully maneuver the situation. A case example can highlight the intricacy involved in self-disclosure.

CASE STUDY 4

Alex is a CEO of a well-known technology firm. He is professionally successful and is a devoted husband and father to his three kids. The reason Alex came in for therapy is to work on issues related to sex with his wife. Alex was in his early forties and sex had all but disappeared from the relationship five years prior. Alex was focused on his career and was fairly busy; however, at night, when home, he would spend an exorbitant amount of time on his computer, looking up porn sites and chatting with women from other countries looking for sexual encounters over the Internet. Alex was too ashamed to admit to himself or his wife that sex had become a major issue in the relationship and spent many months agonizing in therapy over his behaviors on the Internet. Alex did not spend much time discussing his children in therapy and primarily devoted time to his emotional issues and lack of a sex life with his wife. In fact, whenever the subject of his kids did come up in therapy, Alex worked hard to steer the conversation in another direction and focus on sex issues as much as possible.

This experience falls in line with an area therapists call resistance. A therapist knows that if any good therapy is to be done, resistance has to be addressed. At times, when working with a patient, it is possible to discern what hides behind words and at other times, the emotional world of a patient stays obscure. A therapist almost has a sense of being drawn into a battle, where the opponent tries to outsmart the other with certain moves. Experiencing this level of frustration is difficult on the part of a treating clinician, but becomes crucial to a successful therapeutic outcome. The battle has to be resolved in favor of progress in therapy and thus, a therapist is left with a challenging task of having to work with a patient's resistance. From working with Alex for a few months, the therapist learned that the patient had a difficult childhood and was hesitant to discuss specific issues troubling him. Depending on the specific theoretical framework in use by the therapist, it may not always make sense to delve into the past as it touches on working through a patient's specific set of issues. It does, however, make sense to explore the origin of certain issues, especially if the origin of the problem is rooted in a patient's memory of the past.

Although some clinicians may not agree, in our training as therapists we learn to look at life a certain way. The rules we follow trickle into our therapeutic work. Our patients pick up on those rules and have to enter into a contract to be in therapy to be successful. In other words, therapists understand what is required of the patient to be successful and a patient learns to discuss those things that can potentially mean the difference between success and failure in treatment. The "right" therapist will always define for the patient how resistance can be a roadblock to success, and find a way to work with a patient's resistance to achieve desired results. With encouragement, patients discover how a therapist can help and begin to trust in the safety of the relationship to explore issues that are central to a satisfactory outcome.

The word psychotherapy implies that mental distress has taken place and we go to an expert in the field to alleviate that distress. People go to the doctor to address physical pain and to find the "cure." In much the same way, people visit a psychotherapist to obtain the cure for their mental distress. However, rarely does the word "cure" appear next to the word psychotherapy. If there is no cure, then what would be the point of going to a therapist? Why not just sit at home and talk to a friend?

Freud answered this question years ago when he talked about alleviating mental misery through successful analysis. The idea, of course, was that the rational mind would overtake the irrational, and the patient would see how to get out of her own mental labyrinth of unhappiness. A second claim in the analytical process is that by expressing the "repressed," the patient will be free of the negative energy and have more time for personal fulfillment. Unfortunately, not all counselors and therapists today would embrace Freud's idea of a "cure." However, most therapists would adopt Freud's ideas to fit the needs of modern times. As patients, you do not have to embrace the idea of a medical model by which all illness (physical or mental) can be extracted or cured through medical means. Instead, the therapeutic process can be viewed as a psychoeducational journey by which the patient learns to recognize certain thinking patterns or behaviors, either on the conscious or the unconscious levels, as a pattern that contributed to particular mental distress. This experience can be something that a patient chooses to share with a practicing clinician and learns necessary tools and skills to implement changes that can satisfy one's desire for a good life.

Thus, the process of therapy is likely to be an investigative journey that is explorative in nature. The process can be slow at times, and often many patients feel worse before they feel better. This, in my mind, is precisely why therapy is a more valuable endeavor to working through an individual's issues as opposed to getting things quickly "off the chest" with a friend. The therapeutic encounter teaches patients to reflect on their life experience through a relational dynamic, as well as a psychoeducational approach that provides knowledge on recognizing patterns and tools necessary for change.

CASE STUDY 5

Natasha loves warm and sunny climates and is fond of travel. She is also thinking of leaving her husband, who had "provided a more or less stale environment for her personal growth" as she puts it. Given that she is approaching her forties, she is reluctant to plunge into a divorce; however, she is contemplating a trial separation at the very least. Every single time she is ready to move and find a home of her own, Natasha stalls and continues to stay in her marriage. She describes it as a series of events that prevent her from moving forward (holidays, family obligations, shared finances). The separation continues to be on hold, with Natasha growing ever more frustrated with herself and her husband.

In therapy, when asked about her values, as well as the costs and benefits of separation, Natasha names freedom, independence, and an ability to make her own decisions as the primary reasons for wanting to leave. She finds many excuses for her repetitive behavior and calls herself "practical" in needing time to figure out the logistics. "I cannot just pick up and go on a whim." Natasha is clearly stuck in a loop. The task of a therapist is then not to give advice or sway Natasha in one direction versus another, but to enable her to evaluate her emotional needs, along with the needs of the family, and understand the influences that bind her to the status quo. Natasha can either do it on her own in individual therapy or consider couples work as she recognizes her needs and concerns. A therapist's task is to also encourage Natasha to explore her anxiety with both real and imagined hazards of leaving her marriage and consider if those fears and the associated anxiety are tolerable.

So is change possible? I suppose one could argue that change is possible in a logistical sense, and there is nothing preventing Natasha from renting a house and moving her stuff from one place into another. However, the question still remains, is it the right type of change for her? Is she making the right decision? As it so happens, Natasha did come close once to signing a lease on a house, but did not have the emotional energy to close the deal. Natasha stated many times that her persistence and determination could lead toward finding another rental and an eventual change of address. The patient, however, was worried that she would not necessarily experience the feeling of satisfaction at having made a difficult decision to move on with her life. Instead, she kept dwelling in the fear that she might look back and realize that she had made a mistake and be utterly miserable.

Many critics of psychotherapy would argue that any change that does occur in therapy is slow and the patient may still be on the hook wondering about their decisions. More recent psychotherapeutic practices, however, take a more short-term approach to therapy, taking time to substantiate a healing relationship and encourage the patient to look at learning outcomes and specific measurable gains around change. Patients explore in therapy what they can and cannot tolerate and reassess their fears along the way. Therapy is then based upon a trusting exploration led by the patient into the condition of his life. Natasha may indeed decide to eventually accommodate her present-day reality by only making marginal changes in her behavior. That is her right. The therapy assesses those changes against a patient's primary goals upon initial presentation and if those changes have been met, therapy is then concluded.

Furthermore, many patients present to therapy ashamed of the emotional material that they have to process. This shame stretches and covers their relatives and friends from whom they are hiding secrets for the fear of judgment. Many patients find some safety in discussing and exploring their issues in the confines of a therapy room. For example, a young woman presents with an initial concern to tell her family about a long-standing relationship she has with a married man. She feels that her family should know about this relationship; however, she is hesitant to talk about it given the possible level of shame and judgment that she may experience. The first step in her deliberation is to explore the issue in therapy and deal with the associated distress, guilt, angst, and depression. The patient learns tools to deal with her distress and explores her beliefs in tolerating the judgment from family members.

Before concluding this chapter, I would also like to add a statement about the therapist's role in therapy. A patient's role in relation to her friends, family members, or relatives can be tricky. A friend or a sister may resent a patient's standing within the family unit, or a patient may have had a few challenges carrying on a peaceful relationship with a mother-in-law or a father. Perhaps these everyday interactions have the potential to condition our response to another, foregoing an objective stance. The therapist is relieved of that problem. The act of disclosure belongs to the patient, and the act of the provision of a therapeutic, objective treatment rests with the therapist.

12

THE END OF TREATMENT

I seldom end where I wanted to go, but almost always end up where
I needed to be.

—Douglas Adams

Ending therapy can be just as challenging as beginning it. Endings
elicit a number of responses in patients as much as they do in therapists.
The task that rests with the therapist is to facilitate a smooth termination out of therapy, without attempting to hang on to the patient or
accelerate an impromptu ending. How do you know that you are done
with therapy? Well, to answer that question simply from a cognitive-
behavioral stance is that you are done with therapy when your goals are
met. Generally this process is challenging as it requires the patient to
imagine the future without the weekly sessions. Often, patients may
even experience a feeling resembling panic at having to lose a trusted
and safe relationship. As this feeling appears, the therapist reminds the
patient that the feeling is passing, and it is quite normal to associate the
idea of leaving therapy as having to function alone in the world. This
feeling is not validated by anything else, but a sense of aloneness, at
having to manage the self, with recognition of the fact that an important
relationship has ended. Then the patient reviews other interpersonal
relationships that he has and fosters those relationships with friends,
relatives, and colleagues. Thus, when leaving therapy, the patient takes
the responsibility of managing the self and is now better equipped at
dealing with symptoms and life's issues. For many patients, an ending to

the therapeutic process fosters the next question, such as: "Well, what should I do next?" It is a continued discovery of what one wants that precipitates yet another journey based on changes made in treatment.

Interestingly enough, for the therapist, a satisfactory ending can serve as a form of a reward. Many experience a sense of completion and achievement at having been close by to participate in the process of change with a patient who is moving forward in his journey. The critics of psychotherapy might argue that the entire process is a form of self-indulgence, spending the money for issues that can be resolved in other ways. Frankly, I would argue that point vehemently since therapy is in actuality a difficult process, where a patient may get worse before getting better, and additionally has to work very hard to experience any lasting change. An ending for the patient can be a harbinger of new beginnings, as well as a sense of accomplishment. For the therapist, an ending can be considered a loss, certainly financially with having to find new patients, but also a gain, at skillfully helping another with their life goals.

The word "change" keeps coming up again and again in relation to the psychotherapeutic process. As I reflect on this word now, I would say that the biggest difference between a patient before and post therapy is his ability to conceptualize that change is possible. Many come into therapy stagnant, stuck, and afraid to imagine a different possibility for themselves. Many also wait for some changes to happen to them externally, without applying any effort from within. So therapy very much becomes the driving mechanism, with patients tolerating and embracing change, as well as motivating themselves for any changes in the future.

An additional danger in the therapeutic process is a therapist feeling as if the changes that the patient is making are not the "right" type of changes. An example can be a woman pursuing a change in employment, having no particular skill set or education in the new field area. The patient may feel that her time in therapy has helped her come to a difficult decision and leave her current, unhappy place of employment. This type of change may be difficult for the therapist to tolerate; however, when I discuss change, the change that is acceptable to the patient is the determining change in treatment. A therapist may even feel that there are upcoming conflicts in the future that would need to be addressed by the patient as soon as she ceases therapy. Another scenario is a therapist who would hold on to the relationship, believing that the "acceptable change" cannot really be something that a patient has actually decided to do. Frankly, this could be a matter of countertransference where the treating clinician may need to look into her own issues for why a patient's decision is upsetting to them. The problem here can also be an issue of who really knows best? A therapist may be coming from the point of view of a case conceptualization, understanding of the patient, and the theoretical model in use. Unfortunately, none of this matters when it comes to termination. When a patient is convinced that her therapy goals have been met, the therapist has little choice but to let go and convey to the patient that his door is always open for a future appointment. At closure, the task of any therapist and patient is to simply move forward, with the determination and knowledge that what was learned in therapy will carry some weight when making life decisions or managing symptomatology.

Part II

Being in the Room

13

A FEW CASES

People spend a lifetime searching for happiness; looking for peace. They chase idle dreams, addictions, religions, even other people, hoping to fill the emptiness that plagues them. The irony is the only place they ever needed to search was within.

—Ramona L. Anderson

The stories ahead are clinical cases from my own practice, designed to illustrate to the reader what it might be like to be involved in psychotherapeutic treatment. The stories highlight encounters between a patient and a therapist, defining expectations, goals and challenges behind the private realm of treatment. In this mind frame, the reader experiences versions of actual clinical cases, focusing on glimpses of specific dialogue and personal distress. Each of the two cases is designed to shed light on what anyone thinking of beginning psychotherapy might be experiencing behind closed doors. A disclaimer must be made that a great deal of care went into protecting the confidentiality of patients in the next few pages, and all identifiers have been changed including but not limited to gender, age, diagnosis, and personal circumstances. I am certain that if anyone picked up the book, they would not be able to identify the patient in treatment. The dialogue is fictional and is not a transcript of my sessions held as the therapist. My hope is that these cases will be useful to patients, as far as to give an idea of what to expect in therapy and treatment. As stated earlier, I am a cognitive-behavioral therapist, and the cases are examined through the lens of this particular theoretical framework. As a clinical practitioner in the field, I feel that this book would have been incomplete had I not introduced the heart of psychotherapy—the encounter between a therapist and patient.

John was a twenty-year-old man who after experiencing his first manic episode was hospitalized while attending college. John's professors noted that his behaviors grew increasingly more erratic. Shortly after hospitalization, John went back to live at home with his parents. Both of his parents were employed and financially capable and emotionally available to support John through his recovery period.

John started some counseling sessions while at the hospital, receiving psychoeducation around his diagnosis of bipolar disorder. Initial sessions were quite difficult, with John judging that he did not belong in the hospital and did not need any type of psychiatric care. John especially minded the idea of being stereotyped as a "mental patient." As sessions continued, John agreed to take medication for his disorder, firmly believing that he at least wanted to prevent another manic episode from occurring. When John finally came to see me, he appeared weary of initiating another therapeutic encounter, and stated that he simply wanted to get information on treatment for bipolar disorder.

When I asked John to discuss the symptoms associated with his most recent episode, he flinched saying, "I have told my story plenty of times, so you can just read my hospitalization paperwork." I did not want to alienate John, although my initial reaction was to do just that and tell him to find another therapist. I dug a little deeper and found myself empathizing with my patient, validating him in the fact that perhaps it was an incredibly painful experience to describe his symptoms repeatedly to different clinicians. I also did my best to provide some psychoeducation to John, discussing the possibility that sharing the details of his most recent episode might help resolve some of the unresolved feelings associated with being labeled as a mental patient. With that, John's treatment started, and as he came to experience my office as a safe and nonjudgmental place, he was also more inclined to share the details of his racing mind associated with a manic episode.

John recalled the feelings of being "on top of the world" and imagining that he could do anything if he put his mind to it. John focused on his constant activity level, lack of sleep, and recent spending habits. It became clear from John's initial diagnostic interview that he had become manic due to several all-nighters that he had pulled at school while studying for his exams. His symptoms began to escalate after the third night of being sleep deprived. It was apparent that John could benefit from psychoeducation in our treatment, making sense of some of his prodromal symptoms prior to the episode, as well as conflicts and stressors that could have played a role in precipitating his mania.

With our session progressing, John felt visibly more and more uncomfortable discussing his symptoms without explicitly voicing his concerns. After staying quite for a few seconds, John shared that he was having a hard time with his diagnosis, and what it meant to him now that he was labeled "bipolar." It was important then to focus much of the energy of the session on encouraging John to share his feelings and offer support and empathy for his experience.

Me: It must be difficult for you to cope with all of these new symptoms, while trying to make sense of your life.

John: Yeah, you know, I found myself staying up later and later just to get the studying done and then it all came crashing down.

Me: Did you feel like you started having more energy for work?

John: Yes, it was as if someone had given me all this understanding of the subjects I was taking at the time, and I felt like I understood things like never before.

Me: John, do you remember what your experience was like when you were first getting manic?

John: I remember hearing a lot of noises in my head as well as hearing voices. I also remember screaming and laughing a lot. I read a lot of books and kept ordering more books on Amazon.

Me: Do you remember how your body felt at the time?

John: I was really sore all over my body, but could not quite focus on it, since I felt I had more ideas coming in.

Me: It sounds like there were a number of important things going on that were difficult to take in and understand at that moment, which may have contributed to the manic episode. Out of all the symptoms that you experienced, which were the hardest to deal with? Was all of this unexpected? What did you do after you started hearing noises and voices?

An important piece to this discussion with John was to identify precipitating events that led to his manic episode. Gaining an accurate understanding of the precipitating events helped me know the exact factors responsible for John's episode and more importantly, helped highlight those factors as possible triggers for the next episode. In subsequent sessions, John and I discussed the value of categorizing recent life events as losses, transitions, relationships, and interpersonal communicational stressors to help John learn areas of his life that may have been subject to vulnerability. By identifying areas of emotional vulnerability, John helped decrease his own threshold for new manic episodes.

Despite the horror of his episode, John opened up during our sessions, however, continued to minimize the importance of stress in precipitating his mood disorder episode. John insisted on the fact that his illness was purely biological and he would not be able to contain the next "explosion" if it were to occur again. John's belief about the origin of his disorder made me question if I could help him, which was to be addressed if my patient could be open to modifying his beliefs.

John: I think we are grabbing at straws here. So what if I lost sleep for a few nights in a row? That does not necessarily prove a causal relationship to my manic episode.

Me: I think you bring up an excellent point. I also think that it is unlikely that one single event had caused your mania, and I hope I did not convey that in our past discussions.

John: Which proves my points that the root cause of all of this is biological in nature, right?

Me: I can see some of the benefit of thinking this way, since it puts the responsibility of maintaining the disorder purely on psychopharmacology. However, nothing is purely biological. In fact, research has shown that bipolar disorder has both biological causes as well as environmental causes, such as stress.

John: So am I just supposed to quit school, eliminate all stress and never deal with life again?

Me: I think your thinking around it at this point in time only allows you to consider two options, all or nothing. It is either you are completely stressed or not stressed at all. If you already have a biological predisposition to having these episodes, I am sure that additional stress would have had little effect. The value of discussing these issues is that in the future you may know particular kinds of stress that affect you the most, and how to avoid these stressors, or better manage them once they've occurred.

As I considered whether treatment with John would be successful, I tried to minimize potential obstacles to treatment and persuaded myself that my patient's beliefs were malleable to change. John was not unreasonable to question if one single event had caused his manic episode. Such conclusions are faulty and require a thorough examination. My work with John had a large psychoeducational component, where distinctions had to be made in considering whether a single event can be one of many causes and one of many effects on a developing episode. The point had to be made clear that no one single event had caused mania, but rather a collection of events creating a cumulative stress effect that under normal circumstances might be difficult for a nonbipolar individual to handle.

To my surprise, John made excellent use of therapy; and after just a few sessions we were meeting on the regular basis. John came to every session on time, with a list of questions and issues that were a challenge to him during the week. Sometimes we would focus our sessions on how much he hated living with bipolar disorder, most of all loathing that he would need to be on medication for the rest of his life. Even aside from his symptoms and a diagnostic label, John's reaction to hospitalization was quite traumatic, filled with anger, confusion, sadness, and anxiety. We were making progress and, at the moment, I was John's connection to his own experience. I was certain we had to delve into his trauma and make sense of it together. "I know this is something that you have been struggling with for quite some time. I do not think I recall knowing a single patient that had ever liked being in the hospital. Do you feel at all that the event was somehow unjust and that you should not have been hospitalized?" It was important that I communicate to John that his reactions and feelings were not singular only to him, but many patients had experienced this as well.

> John: I just remember I was in the hospital. I think I was yelling and the next thing I knew several doctors surrounded me, grabbed me and began to take me to some room.

> Me: John, I wonder how accurate our memories are of disorienting and traumatic events. Were there really that many doctors surrounding you? I am sure it was scary to have this many people around you at one time dragging you into a room.

> John: What happened next was even scarier, because I remember waking up several days later, or maybe it was that night, but I had a beard and all these thoughts going through my head.

> Me: I appreciate how vivid your account is of that experience. Your fear comes across even now, weeks later, just talking about it with me.

I sat silently for several minutes trying to give my patient the floor and discuss his hospitalization experience in a frank and vulnerable manner. I did my best to highlight to John his own experience, while gently opening up the possibility that it was an experience that John had lived through, and reached some sort of understanding about. It was an experience that was higher than him that suggested self-consciousness and shame. From the way John was speaking, it was evident that he was trying to make peace with his traumatic hospitalization.

One of the most important principles of therapy is that you can create a session as a miniature exposure to whatever environment a patient has dealt with on the outside. Therapy sessions with John created a way for us to reflect on his experience and how he had chosen to live his live since then. Discussing with John the fact that bipolar disorder is usually a recurrent illness and episodes could come and go over time was a valuable realization. Focusing on how John handled his one episode, remembering, recreating, and tolerating the associated fears and anxiety was an issue that my patient had to work through.

John walked away from our initial sessions feeling relieved to have been understood and cared for in terms of his basic human experience of being hospitalized. Most importantly, the treatment itself progressed much faster, as my patient was not intimidated by the interventions, and could see the potential benefits of taking a more active role in his own maintenance of the disorder, aside from simply taking medication. John had a beginning sense of the syndrome of bipolar disorder, including some of its symptoms and initial signs. He learned how to recognize when his episodes occurred, and as a result alleviate a lot of anxiety about the future and recurrent episodes of mania.

After some time, I mused for about a half an hour on the work John and I had done together. Although the treatment itself satisfied me professionally, I had not gotten any appreciation from John that I had been so fervently seeking. Something was amiss and I could not quite place my finger on it. Of course, John had no idea whatsoever as to what I had wanted from him. I could hardly come to terms with my immature needs for appreciation, much less share what I was going through with my patient. So, of course, as time went on, all these thoughts and sentiments of mine remained hidden, until something happened during one of our sessions together where I discovered the crucial ingredients that were missing in my therapy with John.

Once we worked through some of John's conflicts surrounding the trauma at the hospital, the overwhelming sadness that my patient felt signaled the beginning of acceptance. I discovered in sessions that John was grieving over the lost hopes, dreams, and aspirations he once had for himself prior to the changes he made to accommodate his mental illness. John's grieving process helped him get past his denial and accept that he may have to carve out a different life for himself. If I had to write my summary of our one-hour session together, I would choose to focus on two conversations with John, processing and grieving over the loss of his former self.

John: I am hopeless, because I feel like everything that we have talked about implies that everything that I had ever wanted for myself is now lost! There is so much that I had planned and now it seems that I have to resign myself to a life of sedation, because I have to focus all my energy on keeping stress at bay.

Me: John, I want to caution you here, because "everything" is a big word. Do you think we can make a distinction right now between what you have to give up for now, in the immediate future, and what you will have to give up in the long term?

John: I want to be able to finish my school, graduate and find a full-time job. I feel as though I will be behind everyone else if I do not push myself right now.

Me: I can see that not being in school right now is very upsetting to you and I want to validate these feelings that you are experiencing. I also think that just because you are feeling a bit better right now and wanting to push yourself to finish up classes, it could spell out danger in the long run. You have been out of the hospital for a few months and are still very fragile.

John: Well if I am so fragile, why did I get released from the hospital then?

Me: I think you are asking a very broad question here and it could be an issue with our short-term hospitalization system. I would rather not waste the hour discussing this topic, but rather focus on how you could reenter your life gradually, adjusting to the new circumstances.

After approximately half an hour of therapy, John's depression turned to the subject of his lifelong dream to become a neurosurgeon. John's bipolar disorder loomed as a major barrier between his dream and his new life. "Do you think I will ever be able to fulfill my dream?" I heard John ask in a low voice.

Me: Possibly. However, I think the question you really want to ask me is whether you can still allow yourself to dream, have goals, and certain needs. What you want to ask me is whether you can do all the things that you had planned for yourself. I think it is an excellent question to think about and my opinion is that you not only should, but must figure out a way to fulfill all of your life's goals. In fact, many successful, creative people were diagnosed with bipolar disorder.

John: So you think it is still possible for me to become a surgeon even with this label?

Me: Yes. However, I do not want for you to plan too far into the future since some decisions that you make now will affect those that you make later on. As much as I want to devote our time to long-term planning, I would rather focus on the next few months, until you are stabilized enough to decide for yourself whether medicine is the right career path for you.

In this exchange, it was important for me to validate my patient's desire to see himself as separate from his diagnostic label. Moreover, it is always helpful to encourage patients to distinguish short-term versus long-term goals and focus on what can be done in the "now" versus "later." Short-term planning allows John to have a greater sense of control over his decision-making abilities in the future. It is common for patients to idealize and reminisce over the self that they had lost prior to experiencing a manic episode, and it is a fine line to walk for a clinician to challenge what a patient can do, and allow that patient to find some continuity between his former and current self. This challenge subsides with time, and as patients reach a mature self-understanding, bridging the gap between what they can and cannot do becomes easier and clearer.

Accepting a psychiatric diagnosis means accepting being different. In John's case, accepting a psychiatric diagnosis meant that at some point he would have to deal with the uncomfortable feeling of telling his friends, girlfriend and boss about his symptoms or even worse, hospitalization. John's therapy took on a new turn, when he told me one day that people in his life would reject or avoid him once they "knew his diagnosis." John feared that he would be fired from his job at the university and his girlfriend would break up with him. For these reasons, along with some others, John insisted on perpetuating the myth that his illness was not real, and that his manic episode was a one-time occurrence.

John's fear of stigmatization was quite real and quite relevant in today's world. In my experience, many patients fear being stigmatized for mental illness, and anticipate negative repercussions in their work and family lives. John's fear had to be addressed, however, the subject of stigma is a broad and challenging one to tackle. The problem is best discussed around a specific interpersonal relationship, such as the patient's relationship with his employer that can then help him break the issue down into several smaller pieces. I started the session by asking John three questions to get him thinking about his dilemma: "Whom do you tell about your mental disorder?" "Do you have to necessarily share everything with them, including details that are especially difficult to remember, much less voice to someone else?" and "What is the likelihood that these persons will respond negatively to what you have to say?"

Me: This is quite a difficult subject and I appreciate your willingness to discuss it in session. I think it is important to remember that there is no tried and true formula for self-disclosure. Everyone has to find their own way of sharing this information with the people that are important to them. John, how do you feel about self-disclosure, and when you say you want to self disclose, is there a specific person that you have in mind?

John: Specifically, I have been having a hard time figuring out what I am going to say to my boss when I get back to school. I haven't been to work in almost two months and just have no idea how to address the issue.

Me: Well, let's think through this one. From what you know about him, does he appear like a judgmental person to you?

John: Now that you ask, I have to say no. He is very strict, however, I would not go as far as to label him "judgmental."

Me: Can you think of anyone else in your office that has been out for a lengthy period of time?

John: I can think of one person who has been out and when she came back, she shared with everyone that she had been out due to a death in the family.

Me: Can you remember how your boss reacted to her absence and then explanation?

John: He was actually very understanding and offered my colleague more time off if she needed to take it.

Me: So it sounds like he may not be as judgmental as you fear him to be.

John: Well, I guess I just don't know how he would react to an employee with a mental illness.

Me: I can see how you would place mental illness in a different category however, much like anyone else, I believe your boss could benefit from some education around the issue. You might choose to share with him certain information, but leave out certain gory details of your hospitalization. I think in large part you have to do your own share of destigmatizing the disorder to your boss, so that he is not afraid of the diagnostic label.

Practical manifestations of the issue around stigma are often a good prelude to addressing communication and assertiveness skills with patients. John and I spent a good amount of time in session role-playing and practicing self disclose in different ways. John also benefited tremendously from practicing how much to disclose and how to frame his experience of hospitalization. In preplanning for stress and other circumstantial variants, John was also coached on the importance of taking breaks while at work, renegotiating his work hours to start at a later time in the day and asking for leave around medical appointments. It is generally not a patient's preference to disclose their diagnosis of a mental disorder, however, self-disclosure is a good idea as it helps employers know the nature and extent of the disability to provide special accommodations.

After several months of therapy, John and I had to discuss relapse prevention issues inherent in patients who are feeling better and want to discontinue taking medication. The discussion opens the door to understanding John's feelings about medication and his views on whether he thinks he will be on medication for the rest of his life. I found myself addressing the topic right out of the gate one afternoon, attempting to predict John's likelihood for nonadherence. "Although I can see that you are compliant with treatment right now, I am guessing that at some point you are going to feel much better and consider stopping medication use. It is a common phenomenon, since most patients do not like to be dependent on medications for the rest of their lives, in addition to experiencing side effects. I want to bring up this subject now versus later, so that you can address these feelings when they come up either with me or your psychiatrist before you make the decision to stop taking medication." For most clinicians addressing the subject of relapse is uncomfortable, as if conveying to the patient that they expect him to fail. However, most patients who have been diagnosed with a mental illness and have a hard time accepting the diagnosis have considered discontinuing medication at some point. Addressing the subject in therapy is unlikely to precipitate nonadherence, much like addressing the subject of suicide will not precipitate the actual act. Relapse prevention is an important point of discussion, since it gives clinicians a chance to provide some psychoeducation to their patients. First, it allows the patient to understand the risks inherent with discontinuing medication. Second, it informs the patients that they will most likely have to deal with the side effects of medication use for a long time, so that it prepares them to address the subject with their psychiatrist. Finally, a lack of discussion around relapse prevention is currently the major cause of nonadherence. Some patients benefit simply from knowing the risks they face by discontinuing medication use. In rare cases, the patient or the family may have gotten misinformed about having to take medication for the rest of their lives and look at the situation as a one-time deal only, where they take medication as a booster shot. These patients especially can and do benefit from psychoeducation and preventative maintenance.

John's response to relapse prevention was not uncommon, "I'll take meds up until the point when I start feeling better." His position was clear, he was looking at the medication as a one-time shot. Given my patient's reluctance to accept medication as part of his daily routine, I provided psychoeducation, discussing that most mood stabilizing agents only work after several weeks and his symptoms may escalate into another manic episode before the medication can take full effect. Another point to address with John involved the fact that most patients feel euphoric and good when manic. Patients in that state do not want to dull their experience with medication and are thus unable to make the necessary, hard decisions. John was informed that these are all possible risks that he was running into if he chose to discontinue medication after feeling a bit better.

Moreover, many patients want to discontinue their medications because of legitimate complains about side effects. As is a common scenario, most patients who are taking Lithium or Depakote at times experience nausea, sedation, weight gain, and abdominal pain. Discussing the unpleasant possibility of these side effects with John was therapeutic, as it gave him a chance to be validated in his experience. As a clinician, my job was to point out to John that any medication will have costs. However, most medication will also have benefits and it was up to John to evaluate those costs and benefits. My patient pointed out that it was "weird to him to have been healthy his whole life and now have to take pills." Encouraging John to discuss what exactly it meant to him to take medication every morning was a big part of his work in therapy.

John: Taking medication makes me feel like I am dependent on something, almost defective in some way.

Me: I realize that taking Depakote is a decision that you have to make every day and is also a constant reminder of your mental illness. I think we have discussed at length my position on medication and the importance of taking it daily. With that in mind, I also want to validate your difficult experience at facing these daily reminders of your illness. That cannot be easy for anyone.

John: I feel a great deal of frustration and anger with all of this.

Me: It is almost as if someone took away a certain measure of control from your life and it is infuriating.

It is important to clarify the connection between medication taking and John's perceived lack of control in the situation. This connection had to be highlighted in the process of therapy, but also reframed so that the patient understood that taking a daily pill can also make a difference between a life of emotional stability and a life of internal chaos.

Discussing the various ways in which John had to address and face his resistances was monumental work. My patient had to come to terms with the fact that treatment of bipolar disorder is often an indefinite process. Once our therapy was ending, John and I discussed the possibility that he might have to be back again, whether because of a crisis, desire for a referral or just the need to have a constant therapist. I often wondered about John and how well he was doing once he reentered college in the fall of the following year.

Kate's trauma rendered her helpless. She came to me broken and disconnected, searching for meaning. Rape, battery, and other forms of sexual and domestic violence were part of her life. It was part of her experience and it was overwhelming. Kate was confronted with extremes in helplessness and terror and spent the majority of her life responding to catastrophes. Kate described her experience as though she was "disconnected from the present moment." "I am always mentally and physically organized for another attack from my ex-husband. Total strangers on the street assume his face and I cannot help seeing the world as a terrible place."

I knew from clinical experience that after a traumatic event, the human body goes into a state of permanent alert, regardless of the danger at hand. In this state of hyperarousal, the victim is sensitive to any little stimuli that might activate the senses. Kate endorsed most symptoms of trauma including nightmares, psychosomatic complaints, hyperalertness, and startle reactions. Over time, Kate got away from her perpetrator; however, the physiological phenomena persisted, bringing her into my office ill equipped to lead a life of safety and security. Kate suffered from a combination of generalized anxiety symptoms and specific fears related to her trauma. Her increased arousal persisted not only during waking hours, but also during sleep, resulting in a sleep disturbance. Kate's trauma reconditioned her system, leaving her reliving the events of the last ten years as though they were continually recurring in the present.

Kate's traumatic memory almost arrested her development by its repetitive intrusion into her daily life. It was as if she was dominated by it and struggled to make sense of anything else. Her life became her trauma, and her fixation on it was one of the essential features of post-traumatic stress disorder (PTSD). This dark space in her, where nothing made sense, lived only horror, which was expressed inarticulately in short, enraged sentences filled with betrayal. Traumatic memories lack verbal context, rather they are imprinted in a victim's memory as a series of images and physiological sensations. Survivors will often describe a traumatic memory as a still print. Very often, one particular image stands out from the rest and haunts the victim daily. The intense focus on sensations without a verbal context, gives the traumatic memory an emotionally charged feel. "I remember the tattoo on his forearm. I remember his smell. He beat me so hard one time that I could taste the blood on my lips. I think what still wakes me up at night is the memory of his intense, dark eyes. I wake up screaming." Years later, the verbal expression of those four sentences was all that Kate could convey.

Just as traumatic memories were impairing Kate's existence, her traumatic dreams shared similar fragmented features of her horror. They often included fragments of the traumatic event in the exact form, with very little deviation from what had happened in reality. Kate described experiencing the nightmares with intense immediacy, as if the event was occurring in the present. The traumatic memories can also occur in stages of sleep where people do not usually experience dreams, thereby altering a person's sleep cycle as well as neurophysiological functioning. Kate shared that the small, seemingly insignificant environmental cue could always be perceived as a sign of attack by her, giving rise to extreme reactions.

Kate relived her trauma not only in her waking life and through dreams, but also through her behaviors. Kate recalls that in her fervent attempt to change the outcome of her trauma, she found herself being reckless when driving. "I was going out to meet some friends and while on my way there I noticed that this black Volvo next to me was attempting to cut me off from a nearby lane. I saw that the driver was male with features similar to my ex-husband. I said to myself at that moment that there is no way that I would allow him to cut me off. Just like that, two seconds later we collided and I was involved in a car accident." That accident is exactly what brought Kate to my office several months later. "I knew that how I reacted to that driver was dangerous. I also knew that he activated my issues from the abuse. At that time I realized that I needed to deal with my anger and confront my trauma, because if I didn't, I could be found dead somewhere in the next few months."

The changes in consciousness are at the heart of trauma and are yet another symptom of PTSD. At times, triggering situations can provoke rage and pain, forcing the person to lash out and be reckless as was the case with Kate. However, at other times, triggering situations can also leave someone feeling helpless, numb, and detached. The victim may still continue to register a dangerous situation but not react. Perceptions may be distorted, with partial loss of feeling or sensation in the body. Particularly troubling for patients is when there is a time loss, when a traumatic memory is aggravated and the person may feel as though the event is happening outside of his body. These events are generally coupled with feelings of profound numbness and disorientation.

Kate shared in session that she never experienced feelings of numbness or dissociation; however, she did state that she attempted to create similar effects by using alcohol. For my patient, alcohol use allowed her to phase out memories of terror and helplessness and take some comfort in suppressing her flashbacks, albeit dangerous to her health and well-being. The literature on trauma is clear that many patients compound their problems by getting dependent on drug or alcohol use. In fact, veterans are far more likely to develop a dependence on street drugs or alcohol after returning home from war. Although drug use may be an adaptive strategy in the short term, allowing victims to forget and avoid any horrid memories, in the long term, drug use also prevents integration of traumatic events necessary for healing. Thus, more often than not, patients with PTSD are likely to be paralyzed into inaction, not knowing how to keep the painful memories from entering everyday awareness.

Perhaps the most troubling and the most difficult aspect of trauma is that patients lose a sense of self. Traumatic events call into question all human relationships, as well as a sense of security, safety, and self-development. When everything is shattered, victims generally lose themselves in their trauma. Patients are prone to shame, doubt. In the aftermath of traumatic events, survivors doubt everything they see and touch, including themselves. In Kate's case, the damage to her sense of family was particularly severe, as the events from her past involved a betrayal from the person who was closest to her—her husband. After years of abuse, Kate exhibited not only the classic, identifiable symptoms of PTSD, but also grief, disruption in relationships, and chronic depression. Her lost sense of self was a source of much sadness.

Similarly, because Kate's trauma involved a close personal relationship, she was having a hard time letting other people into her life, while concurrently desperately trying to latch onto any man who might provide her with a sense of trust and safety. The fear of traumatic events in her life intensified her need for a protective attachment. Her life became a seesaw of anxious withdrawal from men, followed by a fervent need to connect. In Kate's words, her trauma kicked away any solid ground that her sense of self was rooted in. "It was very clear to me that I was losing control and I had never been so frightened in my life. I felt like I was alone in my nightmare and, what is worse I had to relive the nightmare in my dreams. I was terrified of forming another relationship with someone, and terrified of being completely alone." Kate's self-esteem was damaged greatly by her experiences of humiliation and helplessness. Her capacity to form relationships was compromised by contradictory and intense feelings of attachment as well as fear. "The person that I used to be is no longer here. The Kate that I knew is gone."

The core experiences of Kate's trauma were disempowerment and disconnection from everyone in her life. Recovery therefore was based on two factors: rebuilding the sense of self through empowerment and establishing new connections in her life. Recovery took the form of reshaping, and reshaping involved a recreation of the psychological features of development that were damaged during the trauma. The features that are frequently damaged are trust, safety, initiative, intimacy, and a sense of self. In the initial stages of treatment it was important enough to convey to Kate that she had to be the author of her own recovery. Other people who were in her life that could offer support and a friendly ear could only do so much. I, as a therapist, could only do so much. Kate had to take the initiative for her own choices and behaviors as opposed to me telling her in session what she should do. This would only further undermine any treatment, since I would be in a position similar to her perpetrator where I would try to control her in some way.

The therapy relationship is unique in several aspects as it touches on treating a patient who had experienced trauma. There is the purpose of promoting recovery of course. However, the tricky part is establishing a type of relationship that would promote and restore the patient's sense of control. By virtue of the therapist and patient relationship, the patient comes to the therapist and submits to be assisted and taught. Feelings of dependence and involuntary helplessness are inevitably aroused. This makes the role of the therapist a very difficult one. It then becomes the therapist's responsibility to confer upon the patient the sole purpose of recovery, reiterating the importance of the patient taking charge of his health. In entering the relationship with Kate, I had to promise to help her regain her sense of self, and help her find her autonomy once again by remaining objective and allowing her to make decisions in treatment. I had to make sure that my role was both psychoeducational as well as relational, fostering both insight in my patient, as well as developing an empathetic, genuine connection.

By the nature of Kate's diagnosis, her emotional responses to our therapy had a characteristic type of transference reaction common in many patients suffering from PTSD. My patient's experience of help-lessness and terror trickled into our sessions the moment she walked through the door. Being unable to stand up for herself, crying for help, and feeling utterly abandoned is something that Kate had to address in her work. However, the greater her conviction of helplessness, the more she felt like she needed to give away all of her power to me, the official savior. This fantasy of feeling protected from her trauma is something that helped Kate relieve her trauma. At one point in the session Kate remarked how "frightening it was for her to go into her private nightmare, and how safe she felt having me there to guide her through it." This road can be a slippery one for the treating clinician, as there may come a time in therapy where the therapist fails to live up to the patient's idealized expectations of the designated "savior" role. This idealization serves a protective purpose for the patient, but exposes the therapist to weather the storm when a mistake is made and there exists no room for flaws in the patient's mind. I had to confront Kate's ideal-ization of me as the rescuer in her head and had to deliver a response touching on her need for control. "It must be so frightening to have to put so much faith into the hands of one person. What happens to your faith when you are no longer able to control the person you have en-trusted with all that power?" Though Kate felt desperate to place her recovery in someone else's hands, her entering the therapeutic relation-ship in such a fragile state would inevitably lead to more disappoint-ment and anger. Many traumatized people feel similar feelings of need-ing a rescuer however, as the wounds begin to open in treatment, it is important that the victim feels some semblance of control, and is not further reduced to have to give up more power.

Trauma work is difficult for the therapist as well. It is powerful and infectious. Working with Kate through her abuse, I found myself feel-ing overwhelmed. To a degree, I felt the same anger, despair, and helplessness as my patient. The most difficult part of the work was identifying with Kate's profound sense of loss, grief, and sadness. For days, I would find myself taking on the sadness and swimming in the anguish described by Kate during our sessions. As I found out later in my own supervision, working with trauma victims requires a great deal of balance, since going into the depths of despair with someone can create an atmosphere of being at a funeral. When I caught myself embracing Kate's grief, I tuned into how we could deepen our connection by simply stating aloud what was happening to me in the room, and finding a natural sense of humor and affection for the moment. The alliance and the empathy developed with time, as both Kate and I did the work required to achieve recovery. It was a collaborative artwork of commitment, attunement, and respect.

From the onset, I placed an importance on creating safety in my work with Kate. Trauma had robbed her of a sense of power and control, and the guiding principle in recreating safety involves restoring power and control back to the patient. This task may seem simple, however, is incredibly challenging and takes precedence over anything else that happens in treatment. If the patient does not feel an adequate amount of power and control within the therapeutic relationship, no amount of therapeutic work will possibly help engage the patient in the treatment process. Kate felt unsafe in her body and in her life. Her relational context to other people was disrupted, perturbing her sense of self. The type of safety I was responsible for creating had to touch all the critical aspects of her being. This included the use of medication in order to address some of her more severe symptoms of PTSD, such as hyperarousal. Moreover, the use of cognitive and behavioral strategies in sessions helped log her symptoms as well as coping responses to adequately manage those symptoms. Kate also had to define how to manage difficult situations and develop concrete plans for safety. Finally, Kate learned how to cultivate healthy relationships with others, mobilizing her support system and calling upon all of the self-help organizations available in her area to address her social welfare, mental health, and legal needs.

Safety work with Kate also included focus on body control. Issues involving maintenance of basic needs such as sleep, hygiene, exercise, food, and management of self-destructive behaviors. In Kate's case of recent trauma, her injuries demanded medical attention. After Kate created safety and obtained control of her body, our sessions began to involve work around establishment of a safe living environment, taking into account anything that might have endangered my patient in any way. Because it was particularly challenging to do everything herself, Kate was responsible in mobilizing her social support network to arrange for safe accommodations. These safety concerns were important to address immediately, as the aftermath of a traumatic event at times conditions patients to get used to their abusive situations and gets them into the habit of enduring more abuse.

Safety work also requires mobilization of a social support system and development of a plan for future action. In the aftermath of Kate's trauma, she needed to talk through the degree of threat that still existed for her and to decide if she needed to take any action against her ex-husband. Kate's decision was not necessarily obvious to her and our sessions had to focus on a decisional balance tree, weighing out the pros and cons of her choices in the situation. Kate felt confused, stressed, and ambivalent about doing anything and relied heavily on the opinions of others, including her family members and friends. It was critical in sessions to discuss Kate's control in the matter, to provide some empowerment, and to encourage my patient to start making difficult decisions herself as opposed to relying on the opinion of others. In domestic abuse, the choice to report the abuse to authorities must rest with the survivor. If the survivor does ultimately decide to report the abuser, ideally this opens the door for some resolutions. In reality, however, the legal system can tie up a lot of the survivor's resources, time, and energy. In the worst case scenario, the legal system may even be indifferent to survivors of domestic abuse. Kate had to think through whether the involvement of the legal system would stabilize her life and sense of safety or just invite intrusive traumatic flashbacks. Kate did not take this decision lightly and had to make an informed choice with the full understanding of risks and benefits.

Because Kate's trauma was prolonged over the course of many years, the initial stage of treatment was very difficult as Kate had lost all self-belief and was still somewhat dependent on her ex-husband. Kate had spent many weeks rebuilding her ego, painstakingly remembering the sense of who she used to be before getting married. Kate had to remember what it felt like to take initiative, make plans for the future, and exercise her own judgment independent of the judgment that others may have had around her. In the process of reestablishing safety,

Kate systematically learned to enhance her sense of competency and self-esteem. Moreover, Kate began to develop a sense of trust in our therapeutic relationship, relying on the factors of consistency and my commitment to ensuring safety.

Since the task of the initial therapy stage is long and demanding both on the patient and clinician, it is tempting to bypass this first part altogether and delve into the trauma itself. Kate even insisted at times to jump into the exploratory work by beginning to share graphic details of her abuse, thinking that by sharing her story she would somehow solve her problems and forget her trauma. Kate shared that at the root of her trauma was a belief that by talking about the most gruesome and vile details, she might be able to find a cure and get rid of all the weight of her abuse at once. Patients frequently hold the belief that talking provides a cathartic release, imagining that by getting everything out, the slate would be wiped clean, and the patient will be born again. A clinician's role is again dubious, as the patient invites the therapist to share in the details and the therapist is then required to save the patient by way of inflicting pain and asking the patient to continue sharing the story. Because such an approach can stimulate more intrusive symptoms for the patient, my job with Kate was to continue conducting a thorough evaluation to make sure that the safety was in place before exploring traumatic memories. Erring on the side of caution and patient safety, I had to address with Kate her desire and fantasy for a quick and complete recovery. To counter her idea of a "cathartic release," I compared Kate's recovery to a journey that may take months to address. The metaphor of a journey was meant to prepare Kate for our long work together, addressing both the behavioral and psychological dimensions of her trauma. In the end, it was up to both of us to determine when the safety part of our work was in place, and to then embark on the road of remembrance and loss.

In the second stage of recovery, Kate told her story of the trauma. Kate was responsible for telling the story completely, not leaving any detail to the imagination. The reconstruction work is different from just "telling the story" and involves putting into words images and static remembrances of the traumatic memory. In fact, the first time Kate told her story, she appeared unemotional, as if telling facts to a book-keeper. The therapeutic work behind the story encourages the patient to describe the trauma by providing words to the still images frozen in the brain. The basic principles of safety, support, and encouragement still apply in the second stages of the recovery process, however, it is still up to the patient to describe fully the horrors of the past. The therapist plays a role of an active listener, providing the space necessary for the patient to speak the unfathomable. As Kate told her story, the need to provide safety continued to outweigh the need to face the past. Together, we had to decide whether it was safe for Kate to go into the traumatic labyrinths of her mind and reconstruct her trauma. Working with traumatic memories is a delicate balance of encouraging the patient to not avoid the process while concurrently making sure that approaching the memories too fast does not lead to further damage. The decision regarding pace and timing is something that is left up to the patient's discretion with some input from the treating clinician.

Reconstruction work began with Kate recalling events from the past, long before the start of trauma. This provided continuity to the patient's life, restoring a sense of the past separate from the trauma. Kate spent time discussing her goals and dreams before meeting her ex-husband, providing some background as to the person she used to be before she was robbed of her identity. The next step was focusing on the facts of the trauma and simply connecting events in sequential order. I asked Kate to recall her reaction to the events as well as put into words the most horrible and difficult aspects of her trauma. During the reconstruction it was important to incorporate all senses, including what the patient was seeing, hearing, smelling, and thinking. Often, Kate had trouble verbalizing her still images and was asked to draw pictures of what she was remembering. Kate was also asked to remember her physiological responses to the trauma such as weakness in the muscles, pounding of her heart and dryness of her mouth. The ultimate goal for Kate was to be able to put the entire story into words. Everything that Kate drew and remembered had to be communicated in a language that I, the listener, could understand. Simply sharing the facts of the trauma is not healing. Kate had to face her fear by noting and describing all of her emotions, even as it touched on the most bothersome images that were stored in her memory. The description of emotions had to be just as detailed as the other facts of the trauma. Kate was not simply describing the facts of her trauma in therapy, but reliving the trauma as she was describing it. My job was to provide Kate with a sense of the present moment versus past, so that she could easily maneuver between the two states with confidence and safety necessary for the re-experience to take place.

Reconstructing the trauma also means helping the patient find meaning in the trauma. Kate was responsible for finding her voice in sharing what the trauma had taken from her and the damage that it had done to the person that she once was. Kate had many questions to answer for herself and many "whys" to articulate. Her work, however, was not about the "whys" but about the "hows" in that she had to find a way to work through her grief and find out how she might handle her life now that the trauma had left an imprint on it. My position through all of this was as a neutral bystander, validating my patient's experience and aligning myself with her judgments and stance on what had happened. The exploration becomes one of finding some sort of context that is all encompassing: cognitive and emotional. I normalized Kate's responses and helped her put into words the horror and grief that she was experiencing, constructing an interpretation that was congruent with my patient. Kate frequently mentioned how important it was for her to be validated in our sessions, and that it was this validation that kept Kate encouraged to talk through her pain.

While working through her pain, Kate also had to develop a degree of tolerance for uncertainty, as not all events fell into clear cohesion. In the course of the reconstruction, some events continually changed as the missing information kept getting uncovered. This was particularly true for Kate, since she had experienced significant lapses in memory over the years due to continual and frequent abuse history. Both Kate and I had to accept the fact that her story was incomplete and in some instances changed each time she shared it. This can sometimes be unsettling for patients; however, they must learn to live with uncertainty and confusion while exploring the trauma at a pace that is tolerable. In telling her story, Kate gradually began learning how to transform her trauma from that of guilt, shame, anger, and humiliation to survival, resilience, and dignity. Through her work in remembering her pain, Kate began to gradually gain a sense of the person that she once was, transforming a painful memory into a meaningful individual experience.

Because Kate was a survivor of prolonged, repeated abuse, it was not practical for us to approach each individual memory and work with it as a standalone piece of her pain. Her trauma was long, and over the years, incidents had blurred together with only a few particularly memorable foci. Reconstruction of Kate's trauma was largely based on understanding only a few incidents, with the consideration that these few incidents could represent the many that she had experienced. Allowing for one or two incidents to stand in place of many was an effective technique, as it allowed Kate to create her own meaning from the trauma.

Throughout our work together, Kate had to experience the mourning that her trauma had caused. Abuse always brings loss, and the physical and psychological scars are something that every survivor has to face eventually. Kate frequently resisted the mourning piece of her recovery. Her part of staying strong was not giving way to her tears of pain. She refused to cry or express her mourning in words as a way of denying her ex-husband further victory. Kate and I spent many sessions reframing her inability to mourn as something that might give her courage to move forward as opposed to something that could somehow create more humiliation and loss. Every survivor of trauma should mourn and grieve for the loss of what was taken away from them. If a patient does not grieve, it robs him of a critical part of the recovery process. Once Kate understood that her ability to mourn her traumatic loss was an act of courage rather than further submission to her perpetrator, she finally moved toward resolution, forgiveness, and empowerment.

During the process of mourning, Kate had to also come to terms with the fact that she would not be getting even with her ex-husband for what he had done to her. As Kate vented away her feelings of anger, frustration, and rage, somewhere along the line anger had transformed itself into a sense of control over what she had been through. Her story had taken a different angle, one of survival. Kate was able to transcend her rage and almost willed herself to discover a different type of life. In Kate's case, it was insufficient to continue pointing out that she was the victim and could not help her husband battering. As long as Kate continued to see herself as the victim she would have been unable to take the power back. Acknowledging her own responsibility in staying for as long as she did in an abusive relationship allowed Kate to assume some of the control in the situation. The second stage of remembrance was long and painful. Kate often asked how long she would continue feeling broken and lost. My answer to her was always the same: it might take some time, but surely it will not go on forever.

The third stage of recovery is known as reconnection. After Kate recreated her traumatic past, she was faced with the task of planning for the future. Kate had taken time to grieve over what she had lost during her years of abuse and now had to develop a new sense of self, along with some new relationships. Kate's old ways of thinking had been challenged, leaving her to make new meaning, and establish new faith. In our sessions, Kate frequently spoke of this transition arguably as more challenging than the work she had done prior. It was frightening for her to discover that everything that she once believed in was shattered and she now had to walk into life as if she were an immigrant arriving to a new country. Kate was faced with the challenging task of building a life within a different framework, experiencing both uncertainty and freedom.

During this stage of recovery, Kate understood that she was now capable of creating the type of life and relationships that she desired for herself. Beyond acceptance of this newly found freedom, however, is reevaluation. Kate had to work hard on reassessing her various ways of dealing and coping with social situations, learning to trust new people that entered her life. Kate found herself not only questioning her fear instincts as they touched on new relationships, but also her own role within those new relationships. Kate questioned her traditional acceptance of being a woman in a partnership and playing a subordinate role. Kate learned in the final stages of recovery how her stereotypically feminine attitudes and behaviors can potentially put her at risk in the future. She was also able to revisit her expectations of a dominant, male figure that could render her vulnerable to exploitation in the future. A frank and honest review of Kate's expectations, behaviors, and beliefs had to be undertaken in the last stage of therapy, providing an environment for a nonjudgmental review while ensuring safety.

As Kate recognized her own judgments and assumptions that made her vulnerable to abuse in the past, she was also able to identify sources of social support that could help pave the way into the future. During this time, Kate had to confront the difficult subject of self-disclosure, thinking through how she might self disclose and who she would disclose to. In choosing to keep the secret, survivors of abuse often have to carry the weight of a burden that does not belong to them. Therefore, in my work with Kate, I had to encourage her to break the rule of silence and in so doing renounce the responsibility, guilt and shame that the secret represented. Self-disclosures can be incredibly empowering for the patient if discussed prior in session. Once Kate felt ready to self-disclose to her family about her years of abuse, she also felt prepared to again embrace the power and control that had been taken away from her. At one point in our work, Kate had asked me what would happen if her family renounced her after self-disclosure or somehow denied the truth. In this circumstance, I guided Kate through the exploration of her feelings if self-disclosure for her did not lead to validation. Kate came to the conclusion that for her, self-disclosure would be gratifying enough, and if the family chose to respond with denial or anger then it was on them and not on her. In practice, Kate's disclosure led to validation and she no longer felt intimidated by her family or compelled to keep a secret of this magnitude in the future.

The rest of the time in therapy, Kate focused on recreating and reconnecting with herself after the trauma. As Kate shed away her identity of being the victim, she also shed away parts of herself that felt congruent with her as the victim. This process is challenging, as it asks patients to be able to imagine themselves to be different from what they have known to be true for years. As Kate went through the journey of reconnection, she reported feeling calmer and more at peace with what had happened. At times, she almost felt strange leading a life that was so calm, having been used to feeling on edge and scared for the most part of her days. Kate was able to embrace this new calm life and experience normality for the first time. As Kate recognized and let go of her former self, she was also able to forgive herself for staying in an abusive relationship. Kate was able to express that the damage that she experienced at the hands of her abuser was no doubt traumatic; however, it did not have to be permanent. The more Kate was able to actively engage in rebuilding her life, the more accepting she was of herself when looking back to the memory of her trauma. As this stage of recovery was achieved, Kate felt a renewed sense of pride for everything she had been through and everything she wanted for herself in the future. "I learned how to survive" was Kate's statement during one of her final sessions.

In the last few weeks of our work together, I recommended that Kate join a group for survivors of repeated trauma. The idea behind this recommendation was that while exploring traumatic experiences in a group setting, Kate could share her unique story and the group could give her a source of emotional support and an experience of shared meaning. The group could witness Kate's difficult journey and give personal meaning, as one survivor shares his story with other survivors. Though sharing a personal story may be difficult in an unfamiliar setting, group work has the capacity to bring members strength through dialogue and a strong, shared sense of the terrifying power of abuse. Commonality with other people carries with it all the meanings of recovery: a sense of belonging, safety, and trust. It means taking part in something where a survivor can achieve a feeling of accomplishment for all that had been.

My therapy with Kate eventually ended. Her past was downright ugly, filled with turmoil and fear. Some attacks are unforgettable. And for many, there can be no greater injury. Though challenging, Kate's road to recovery was her tribute to the power of what a single healing relationship can do to the human spirit. Kate was taught that stabilizing her world and speaking the truth ultimately brought her peace of mind and freedom from the constraints of the past. Kate achieved that peace and freedom and finally focused on the rest of her life.

14

CONCLUSION

There is no real ending. It's just a place where you stop the story.

—Frank Herbert

You may have noticed by now that this book is not about me or the latest clinically approved methods of treatment for any single mental disorder. This book is filled with thoughts based on my clinical training and experience on what would make for a helpful treatment experience of any person thinking about beginning therapy. I could not have written this book when I first began counseling patients, because almost everything I read was from the point of view of the treating clinician. I always intellectually knew that it was not about the therapist, but it was difficult to swallow since almost every book was written from a perspective of someone treating versus someone being treated.

An essential part of being a good clinician is the journey of accepting self-limitations, opening up to feedback and at times even criticism. Being open to feedback requires patients to actually have the necessary knowledge on what to expect when seeking professional therapeutic help. Unfortunately, many books written in the past twenty years have focused almost exclusively on what therapists do in therapy versus how to be an informed patient in therapy. The latter is assumed and is somehow being handled, yet this is not always the case. Most people, when entering therapy, know very little in regards to what to expect in treatment. Being in therapy for most people is not on the to-do list and is mostly a vague and distant concept. In line with the same attitude, therapy becomes something that patients have learned to accept as "done on to them" as opposed to "with them."

I prefer to think of the process of being in therapy as a collaboration between two parties. This is why over the years I have shifted my perspective from self-discovery and learning the latest and greatest techniques to sharing this experience with my patients and sending them out to inform themselves first before the burden of the responsibility of treatment is blindly placed into my hands. The key to successful treatment is mutual awareness, knowledge, and feedback. In writing this book, I chose to focus on the patient, which is why I invite you to do further research into the process of psychotherapy before signing up for treatment.

After all the cautions, warnings, and red flags, why would you still want to go into treatment? Truth is, despite all the risks and challenges, being an informed patient in treatment can be an incredibly rewarding and meaningful experience. Although probably a difficult process to navigate both intellectually and emotionally, therapy can offer people a place to open up and simultaneously stretch their own boundaries of trust, safety, and perception. When patients ask me why I became a therapist, which I admit can at times be draining, I respond by saying that I believe in the process of change and that psychotherapy can be a vehicle for that change. My fondest memory is of a session I had with a young lady seeking treatment for depression. After a long time of schooling she was finally able to commit to a process of building her career, which she unfortunately did not find very rewarding. When she mentioned to me one day that her life had become one giant spiral of mistakes, I suggested that she bring to our next session items in her life that she did not consider a mistake.

Sitting on the couch next session was my patient with a photo album. Nervously looking over, my patient began by describing the memories she had as a toddler, her then house on the East Coast, expressing joy and pride at her younger sister just graduating from college. She told me how difficult it was for her growing up without her mother and having to be an adult figure for her younger sister. Both beautiful and deeply troubled, the memory of my patient's face as she was clutching the photo album is something that continues to stand out in my mind to this day. Patients working hard to figure out what would bring them hope and a deeper connection to who they are empowers me to believe in the value of my work. These are rich and satisfying rewards not only for me as a clinician but also my patients, as they find their own personal meaning in the work that they do in treatment.

Ironically, as challenging as the process of therapy can be, it can also deepen further with patients willing to discover and enter more intensely into a dialogue with their therapists, their own lives and with themselves. Many find it gratifying in the end to courageously open up to a stranger and be willing to experience what life can be like for them through this process of cognitive and behavioral change. The trick is remembering to look and do the research in the beginning, be open and ready to give feedback during, and find the willingness to face life with changes afterward.

NOTES

2. THEORIES OF PSYCHOTHERAPY

1. Gregory J. Novie, "Psychoanalytic Theory," in *Counseling and Psychotherapy Theories and Interventions*, 4th ed., eds. David Capuzzi and Douglass Gross (Upper Saddle River, NJ: Prentice Hall, 2007), 87–88.

2. Seymour Fisher and Roger Greenberg, *The Scientific Credibility of Freud's Theories and Therapy* (New York: Basic Books, 1977).

3. Alfred Adler, "The Fundamental View of Individual Psychology," *International Journal of Individual Psychology* 1 (1935): 4.

4. Alan Miliren, Timothy D. Evans, and John F. Newbauer, "Adlerian Theory," in *Counseling and Psychotherapy Theories and Interventions*, 4th ed., eds. David Capuzzi and Douglass Gross (Upper Saddle River, NJ: Prentice Hall, 2007), 157–158.

5. Miliren, Evans, Newbauer, "Adlerian Theory," 140.

6. Mary Lou Bryan Frank, "Existential Theory," in *Counseling and Psychotherapy Theories and Interventions*, 4th ed., eds. David Capuzzi and Douglass Gross (Upper Saddle River, NJ: Prentice Hall, 2007), 165.

7. Frank, "Existential Theory," 184.

8. Richard J. Hazler, "Person-Centered Theory," in *Counseling and Psychotherapy Theories and Interventions*, 4th ed., eds. David Capuzzi and Douglass Gross (Upper Saddle River, NJ: Prentice Hall, 2007), 193–194.

9. Hazler, "Person-Centered Theory," 210–211.

10. Uwe Strumpfel and Clark Martin, "Research on Gestalt Therapy," *International Gestalt Journal* 27, no. 1 (2004): 10–11.

11. Melinda Haley, "Gestalt Theory," in *Counseling and Psychotherapy Theories and Interventions*, 4th ed., eds. David Capuzzi and Douglass Gross (Upper Saddle River, NJ: Prentice Hall, 2007), 228–231.

12. Haley, "Gestalt Theory," 238.

13. Cynthia R. Kalodner, "Cognitive-Behavior Theories," in *Counseling and Psychotherapy Theories and Interventions*, 4th ed., eds. David Capuzzi and Douglass Gross (Upper Saddle River, NJ: Prentice Hall, 2007), 247–248.

14. Kalodner, "Cognitive-Behavior Theories," 259.

15. Robert E. Wubbolding, "Reality Therapy Theory," in *Counseling and Psychotherapy Theories and Interventions*, 4th ed., eds. David Capuzzi and Douglass Gross (Upper Saddle River, NJ: Prentice Hall, 2007), 291–293.

16. Wubbolding, "Reality Therapy Theory," 294.

17. Wubbolding, "Reality Therapy Theory," 295–305.

18. Wubbolding, "Reality Therapy Theory," 308.

19. David Lawrence, "The Effects of Reality Therapy Group Counseling on the Self-Determination of Persons with Developmental Disabilities," *International Journal of Reality Therapy* 23, no. 2 (2004): 9–10.

20. Wubbolding, "Reality Therapy Theory," 307.

21. Ann Vernon, "Rational Emotive Behavior Therapy," in *Counseling and Psychotherapy Theories and Interventions*, 4th ed., eds. David Capuzzi and Douglass Gross (Upper Saddle River, NJ: Prentice Hall, 2007), 267–268.

22. Vernon, "Rational Emotive Behavior Therapy," 282–284.

3. INTERVENTIONS IN PSYCHOTHERAPY

1. Rebecca Crane, *Mindfulness-Based Cognitive Therapy* (New York: Routledge, 2009), 3.

2. John D. Teasdale, "Metacognition Mindfulness and the Modification of Mood Disorders," in *Behavioral and Cognitive Psychotherapy* 6 (1999): 150–151.

3. Crane, *Mindfulness Based-Cognitive Therapy*, 51–52.

4. Crane, *Mindfulness-Based Cognitive Therapy*, 81.

5. Crane, *Mindfulness-Based Cognitive Therapy*, 83–90.

6. Shauna Shapiro and Linda Carlson, *The Art and Science of Mindfulness: Integrating Mindfulness into Psychology and the Helping Professions*. Washington, DC: American Psychological Association, 2009), 53.

7. Shapiro and Carlson, *The Art and Science of Mindfulness*, 53–54.

8. Shapiro and Carlson, *The Art and Science of Mindfulness*, 54–55.

9. Shapiro and Carlson, *The Art and Science of Mindfulness*, 55.

10.   Paul E. Flaxman, J. T. Blackledge, and Frank W. Bond, *Acceptance and Commitment Therapy: Distinctive Features* (New York: Routledge, 2011), 5.

11.   Flaxman, Blackledge, and Bond, *Acceptance and Commitment Therapy*, 9.

12.   Flaxman, Blackledge, and Bond, *Acceptance and Commitment Therapy*, 21–22.

13.   Flaxman, Blackledge, and Bond, *Acceptance and Commitment Therapy*, 34–35.

14.   Flaxman, Blackledge, and Bond, *Acceptance and Commitment Therapy*, 36.

15.   Flaxman, Blackledge, and Bond, *Acceptance and Commitment Therapy*, 37.

16.   Flaxman, Blackledge, and Bond, *Acceptance and Commitment Therapy*, 39.

17.   Flaxman, Blackledge, and Bond, *Acceptance and Commitment Therapy*, 41–43.

18.   Steve C. Hayes, "Association for Contextual Behavioral Sciences," *Outcome Studies* 35 (2010): 1–26. Accessed February 13, 2012, www.contextualpsychology.org/analogue_studies_component_studies_and_correlational_studies.

4. ASKING THE "RIGHT" QUESTIONS

1.   Michael Lambert, Jason Whipple, David Vermeersch, David Smart, Eric Hawkins, Stevan Lars Nielsen, and Melissa Goates. "Enhancing Psychotherapy Outcomes via Providing Feedback on Client Progress: A Replication." *Clinical Psychology and Psychotherapy* 9 no. 2 (2002): 99–101.

5. THE VULNERABLE PATIENT

1.   Danny C. K. Lam, *Cognitive Behavior Therapy: A Practical Guide to Helping People Take Control* (New York: Routledge, 2008), 8–13.

2.   Maurizio Pompili, Iginia Mancinelli, and Roberto Tatarelli. "Stigma as a Cause of Suicide." *The British Journal of Psychiatry* 183, no. 2 (2003): 173–174.

3.   Jill Rachbeisel, Jack Scott, and Lisa Dixson. "Co-occurring Severe Mental Illness and Substance Use Disorders," *Psychiatric Services* 50, no. 11 (1999): 1427-1434.

4. Lisa Barney, Kathleen Griffiths, Helen Christensen, and Anthony Jorm. "Exploring the Nature of Stigmatising Beliefs about Depression and Help-Seeking: Implications for Reducing Stigma." *BMC Public Health* 9, no. 61 (2009): 4–7.

6. BEHIND PSYCHIATRIC DRUGS

1. Jacqueline A. Sparks, Barry L. Duncan, Cavid Cohen, and Davido O. Antonuccio, "Psychiatric Drugs and Common Factors: An Evaluation of Risks and Benefits for Clinical Practice," in *The Heart and Soul of Change*, 2nd ed., eds. Barry L. Duncan, Scott D. Miller, Bruce E. Wampold, and Mark A. Hubble (Upper Saddle River, NJ: Prentice Hall, 2007), 199.

2. Mary Larson, Kay Miller, and Kathleen Fleming, "Treatment with Antidepressant Medications in Private Health Plans," *Administration Policy in Mental Health and Mental Health Services Research* 34 (2007): 116–126.

3. M. Thase, J. Greenhouse, E. Frank, C. Pilkonis, and P. Hurley, "Treatment of Major Depression with Psychotherapy or Psychotherapy-Pharmacotherapy Combinations," *Archives of General Psychiatry* 54 (1997):1009–1015.

4. Sparks el al., "Psychiatric Drugs and Common Factors," 203.

5. Sparks et al., "Psychiatric Drugs and Common Factors," 203–204.

6. Carmen Moreno, Gonzalo Laje, Carlos Blanco, Huiping Jiang, Andrew Schmidt, and Mark Olfsen, "National Trends in the Outpatient Diagnosis and Treatment of Bipolar Disorder in Youth," *Archives of General Psychiatry* 64 (2007): 1034.

7. William Cooper, Patrick Arbogast, Hua Ding, Gerald Hickson, Catherine Fuchs, and Wayne Ray, "Trends in Prescribing of Antipsychotic Medications for U.S. Children." *Ambulatory Pediatrics* 6, no. 2 (2006): 80–81.

8. Sparks et al., "Psychiatric Drugs and Common Factors," 208.

9. David Willman, "Stealth Merger: Drug Companies and Government Medical Research." *Los Angeles Times*, December 7, 2003, A1.

10. Daniel Safer, "Design and Reporting Modifications in Industry-Sponsored Comparative Psychopharmacology Trials," *Journal of Nervous and Mental Disease* 190 (2002): 585.

7. INDIVIDUAL VERSUS GROUP THERAPY

1. Irvin D. Yalom, *Inpatient Group Psychotherapy* (New York: Basic Books, 1983),

25–36.

2. Louis R. Ormont, *The Group Therapy Experience* (New York: St. Martin's Press, 1992), 3.

3. Ormont, *The Group Therapy Experience*, 27–50.

4. Ormont, *The Group Therapy Experience*, 83–98.

8. MEASURING THERAPEUTIC OUTCOMES

1. Michael Lambert and Ben Ogles, "The Efficacy and Effectiveness of Psychotherapy," in *Bergin and Garfield's Handbook of Psychotherapy and Behavior Change*, 5th ed., ed. Michael Lambert (New York: Wiley, 2004), 139–193.

2. Michael Lambert, "Yes, It Is Time for Clinicians to Routinely Monitor Treatment Outcome," in *The Heart and Soul of Change*, 2nd ed., eds. Barry L. Duncan, Scott D. Miller, Bruce E. Wampold, and Mark A. Hubble (Upper Saddle River, NJ: Prentice Hall, 2007), 251–256.

3. Ann Marie Brannan, Craig Ann Heflinger, and Michael Foster. "The Role of Caregiver Strain and Other Family Variables in Determining Children's Use of Mental Health Services." *Journal of Emotional and Behavioral Disorders* 11, no. 2 (2003): 77–91.

4. John C. Norcross, "The Therapeutic Relationship," in *Heart and Soul of Change*, 2nd ed., eds. Barry L. Duncan, Scott D. Miller, Bruce E. Wampold, and Mark A. Hubble (Washington, DC: American Psychological Association, 2010), 113–135.

9. ADVANTAGES AND DISADVANTAGES OF INSURANCE

1. John C. Norcross, "The Therapeutic Relationship," in *Heart and Soul of Change*, 2nd ed., eds. Barry L. Duncan, Scott D. Miller, Bruce E. Wampold, and Mark A. Hubble (Washington, DC: American Psychological Association, 2010), 113–135.

2. John Z. Sadler, "Descriptions and Prescriptions: Values, Mental Disorders, and the DSMs." *Perspectives in Biology and Medicine* 47, no. 1 (2004): 152–157.

3. Ronald J. Comer. *Abnormal Psychology* (New York: Worth Publishers, 2010), 17–21.

4. David Law and Russell Crane, "The Influence of Marital and Family Therapy on Health Care Utilization in a Health-Maintenance Organization," *Journal of Marital and Family Therapy* 26, no. 3 (2000): 281–291.

BIBLIOGRAPHY

Adler, Alfred. "The Fundamental View of Individual Psychology." *International Journal of Individual Psychology* 1 (1935): 1–8.

Barney, Lisa, Kathleen Griffiths, Helen Christensen, and Anthony Jorm. "Exploring the Nature of Stigmatising Beliefs about Depression and Help-Seeking: Implications for Reducing Stigma." *BMC Public Health* 9, no. 61 (2009): 1–8.

Brannan, Ann Marie, Craig Ann Heflinger, and Michael Foster. "The Role of Caregiver Strain and Other Family Variables in Determining Children's Use of Mental Health Services." *Journal of Emotional and Behavioral Disorders* 11, no. 2 (2003): 77–91.

Comer, Ronald J. *Abnormal Psychology.* New York: Worth Publishers, 2010.

Cooper, William, Patrick Arbogast, Hua Ding, Gerald Hickson, Catherine Fuchs, and Wayne Ray, "Trends in Prescribing of Antipsychotic Medications for U.S. Children." *Ambulatory Pediatrics* 6, no. 2 (2006): 79–83.

Crane, Rebecca. *Mindfulness-Based Cognitive Therapy.* New York: Routledge, 2009.

Fisher, Seymour, and Roger Greenberg. *The Scientific Credibility of Freud's Theories and Therapy.* New York: Basic Books, 1977.

Flaxman, Paul E., J. T. Blackledge, and Frank W. Bond. *Acceptance and Commitment Therapy: Distinctive Features.* New York: Routledge, 2011.

Frank, Mary Lou Bryant, "Existential Theory," in *Counseling and Psychotherapy Theories and Interventions*, 4th ed. Edited by David Capuzzi and Douglass Gross, 164–188. Upper Saddle River, NJ: Prentice Hall, 2007.

Haas, M., A. Unis, and M. Copenhaver. "Efficacy and Safety of Risperidone in Adolescents with Schizophrenia." Poster session presented at the 160th Annual Meeting of the American Psychiatric Association, San Diego, CA, May 2007.

Haley, Melinda. "Gestalt Theory," in *Counseling and Psychotherapy Theories and Interventions*, 4th ed. Edited by David Capuzzi and Douglass Gross, 216–242. Upper Saddle River, NJ: Prentice Hall, 2007.

Hayes, Steven C. "Association for Contextual Behavioral Sciences," *Outcome Studies* 35 (2010): 639–665. Accessed February 13, 2012, www.contextualpsychology.org/analogue_studies_component_studies_and_correlational_studies.

Hazler, Richard J. "Person-Centered Theory," in *Counseling and Psychotherapy Theories and Interventions*, 4th ed. Edited by David Capuzzi and Douglass Gross, 189–215. Upper Saddle River, NJ: Prentice Hall, 2007.

Kalodner, Cynthia R. "Cognitive-Behavior Theories," in *Counseling and Psychotherapy Theories and Interventions*, 4th ed. Edited by David Capuzzi and Douglass Gross, 243–265. Upper Saddle River, NJ: Prentice Hall, 2007.

Keck, P., J. Calabrese, R. McQuade, W. Carlson, B. Carlson, and L. Rollin. "A Random-ized,Double-Blind, Placebo-Controlled, 26-Week Trial of Aripiprazole in Recently Manic Patients with Bipolar I Disorder." *Journal of Clinical Psychiatry* 67 (2006): 626–637.

Kirsch, Irving, and Guy Sapirstein, "Listening to Prozac but Hearing Placebo: A Meta-Analysis of Antidepressant Medication." *Prevention and Treatment* 1 (1998): 1–16. Ac-cessed February 11, 2011, doi: 10.1037/1522-3736.1.1.12a

Kirsch, Irving, Thomas Moore, Alan Ascoboria, and Sarah Nicholls, "The Emperor's New Drugs: An Analysis of Antidepressant Medication Data Submitted to the U.S. Food and Drug Administration." *Prevention and Treatment* 5 (2002): 10–22. Acessed February 11, 2011, doi: 10.1371/journal.pmed.0050045.

Kushner, S., A. Unis, and M. Copenhaver. "Acute and Continuous Efficacy and Safety of Risperidone in Adolescents with Schizophrenia." Poster session presented at the 54th Annual Meeting of the American Academy of Child and Adolescent Psychiatry, Boston, October 2007.

Lam, Danny C. K. *Cognitive Behavior Therapy: A Practical Guide to Helping People Take Control.* New York: Routledge, 2008.

Lambert, Michael. "Yes, It Is Time for Clinicians to Routinely Monitor Treatment Out-come," in *The Heart and Soul of Change*, 2nd ed. Edited by Barry L. Duncan, Scott D. Miller, Bruce E. Wampold, and Mark A. Hubble, 239–261. Upper Saddle River, NJ: Prentice Hall, 2007.

Lambert, Michael, and Ben Ogles. "The Efficacy and Effectiveness of Psychotherapy," in *Bergin and Garfield's Handbook of Psychotherapy and Behavior Change*, 5th ed. Edited by Michael Lambert, 139–193. New York: Wiley, 2004.

Lambert, Michael, Jason Whipple, David Vermeersch, David Smart, Eric Hawkins, Stevan Lars Nielsen, and Melissa Goates. "Enhancing Psychotherapy Outcomes via Providing Feedback on Client Progress: A Replication." *Clinical Psychology and Psychotherapy* 9, no. 2 (2002): 91–103.

Larson, Mary, Kay Miller, and Kathleen Fleming, "Treatment with Antidepressant Medica-tions in Private Health Plans." *Administration Policy in Mental Health and Mental Health Services Research* 34 (2007): 116–126.

Law, David, and Russell Crane. "The Influence of Marital and Family Therapy on Health Care Utilization in a Health-Maintenance Organization." *Journal of Marital and Family Therapy* 26, no. 3 (2000): 281–291.

Lawrence, David. "The Effects of Reality Therapy Group Counseling on the Self-Determi-nation of Persons with Developmental Disabilities." *International Journal of Reality Ther-apy* 23, no. 2 (2004): 9–15.

Miliren, Alan P., Timothy D. Evans, and John F. Newbauer, "Adlerian Theory," in *Counsel-ing and Psychotherapy Theories and Interventions*, 4th ed. Edited by David Capuzzi and Douglass Gross, 123–163. Upper Saddle River, NJ: Prentice Hall, 2007.

Moreno, Carmen, Gonzalo Laje, Carlos Blanco, Huiping Jiang, Andrew Schmidt, and Mark Olfsen, "National Trends in the Outpatient Diagnosis and Treatment of Bipolar Disorder in Youth." *Archives of General Psychiatry* 64 (2007): 1032–1039.

Norcross, John C. "The Therapeutic Relationship," in *Heart and Soul of Change*, 2nd ed. Edited by Barry L. Duncan, Scott D. Miller, Bruce E. Wampold, and Mark A. Hubble, 57–79. Washington, DC: American Psychological Association, 2010.

Novie, Gregory J. "Psychoanalytic Theory," in *Counseling and Psychotherapy Theories and Interventions*, 4th ed. Edited by David Capuzzi and Douglass Gross, 74–97. Upper Saddle River, NJ: Prentice Hall, 2007.

Ormont, Louis R. *The Group Therapy Experience.* New York: St. Martin's Press, 1992.

Pompili, M., I. Mancinelli, and R. Tatarelli. "Stigma as a Cause of Suicide." *The British Journal of Psychiatry* 183, no. 2 (2003): 173–174.

RachBeisel, Jill, Jack Scott, and Lisa Dixon. *Treatment of Mental Illness and Substance Abuse.* Washington, DC: American Psychiatric Association, 1999.

Ross, Randal G. "New Findings on Antipsychotic Use in Children and Adolescents with Schizophrenia Spectrum Disorders." *American Journal of Psychiatry* 165 (2008): 1369–1372.

Sadler, John Z. "Descriptions and Prescriptions: Values, Mental Disorders, and the DSMs." *Perspectives in Biology and Medicine* 47, no. 1 (2004): 152–157.

Safer, Daniel. "Design and Reporting Modifications in Industry-Sponsored Comparative Psychopharmacology Trials." *Journal of Nervous and Mental Disease* 190 (2002): 583–592.

Shapiro, Shauna, and Linda Carlson. *The Art and Science of Mindfulness: Integrating Mindfulness into Psychology and the Helping Professions.* Washington, DC: American Psychological Association, 2009.

———. *The Art and Science of Mindfulness: Integrating Mindfulness into Psychology and the Helping Professions.* Washington, DC: American Psychological Association, 2009.

Sparks, Jacqueline A., Barry L. Duncan, David Cohen, and Davido O. Antonuccio, "Psychiatric Drugs and Common Factors: An Evaluation of Risks and Benefits for Clinical Practice," in *The Heart and Soul of Change*, 2nd ed. Edited by Barry L. Duncan, Scott D. Miller, Bruce E. Wampold, and Mark A. Hubble, 199–226. Upper Saddle River, NJ: Prentice Hall, 2007.

Stumpfel, Uwe, and Clark Martin. "Research on Gestalt Therapy." *International Gestalt Journal* 27, no. 1 (2004): 9–54.

Teasdale, John D. "Metacognition, Mindfulness and the Modification of Mood Disorders," in *Behavioral and Cognitive Psychotherapy* 6 (1999): 146–155.

Thase, M., J. Greenhouse, E. Frank, C. Pilkonis, and P. Hurley. "Treatment of Major Depression with Psychotherapy or Psychotherapy-Pharmacotherapy Combinations." *Archives of General Psychiatry* 54 (1997): 1009–1015.

Vernon, Ann. "Rational Emotive Behavior Therapy," in *Counseling and Psychotherapy Theories and Interventions*, 4th ed. Edited by David Capuzzi and Douglass Gross, 266–288. Upper Saddle River, NJ: Prentice Hall, 2007.

Willman, David. "Stealth Merger: Drug Companies and Government Medical Research." *Los Angeles Times*, December 7, 2003, A1.

Wubbolding, Robert E. "Reality Therapy Theory," in *Counseling and Psychotherapy Theories and Interventions*, 4th ed. David Capuzzi and Douglass Gross, 289–312. Upper Saddle River, NJ: Prentice Hall, 2007.

Yalom, Irvin D. *Inpatient Group Psychotherapy.* New York: Basic Books, 1983.

INDEX

ABC model. *See* activating event, beliefs, and emotional or behavioral consequences
acceptance, 35
acceptance and commitment therapy (ACT), 34; acceptance in, 35; anxiety controlled by, 37; behavior outcomes and, 38; beliefs and, 35; commitment in, 38; diffusion used in, 36; empowerment from, 42; example of, 35; expectations of, 39; explorative stage during, 41; language and, 37; learning influenced by, 36; premise of, 34, 39; present moment and, 36; randomized controlled trials on, 42; sample session of, 40–41; strategy workability and, 41; therapist's use of, 39; values involved in, 38
accountability, of therapist, 4, 48
ACT. *See* acceptance and commitment therapy
activating event, beliefs, and emotional or behavioral consequences (ABC model), 24
ADAA. *See* Anxiety and Depression Association of America
Adams, Douglas, 113
ADHD. *See* attention-deficit hyperactivity disorder
Adlerian theory, 7; analysis and, 10; anxiety issue example and, 9–10; critics

on, 11; encouragement and, 10
Adult Children of Alcoholics, 67
adverse drug reactions, 63
The Agency for Healthcare Research and Quality, 59
AKQUASI system, 80
alcohol abuse, traumatic event and, 134
Alcoholics Anonymous, 67
Alderian theory, 11
American Psychological Association (APA), 44
Anderson, Ramona L., 119
antidepressant medication: commonality of, 59; efficacy of, 60; placebo compared to, 60; as psychotropic drugs, 59
antipsychotic drugs: child research limitations for, 61; mental illness managed by, 60; side effects of, 61, 130
antistigma campaigns: for mental illness, 55; news stories influencing, 56; research for, 56
anxiety, 19; ACT controlling, 37; Adlerian theory and, 9–10; individual therapy and, 74; psychoanalytical theory and, 9
Anxiety and Depression Association of America (ADAA), 44
APA. *See* American Psychological Association

ABOUT THE AUTHOR

Ilyana Romanovsky is a marriage and family therapist intern specializing in cognitive behavioral therapy. She has extensive experience working with adults, adolescents, and children, focusing on areas of anxiety, depression, social phobia, mood disorders, hoarding, trichotillomania, and dual diagnosis. Ilyana Romanovsky is a professional member of the California Association for Marriage and Family Therapists and is also a member of the Association for Behavioral and Cognitive Therapies. She is currently working in private practice and is a staff clinician with John Muir Behavioral Health in Concord, California.